The Long Goodbye

Also by Suzanne Ross

An Ordinary Person with an Extraordinary God
Spiderwize: Diadem Books, 2010
ISBN10 1907294686
ISBN13 9781907294686

The Long Goodbye

by

Suzanne Ross

SHOSHANNAH MINISTRIES
Walking the walk of dementia with Jesus

DIADEM BOOKS

THE LONG GOODBYE
Copyright © 2021 **Suzanne Ross**

Published by Diadem Books
www.diadembooks.com

ISBN: 9798788414133

MY TRIBUTE TO PETER
– at his funeral.

Peter died and went Home late Tuesday night, 5th March 2018. The Peace that surpasses ALL understanding visibly grew on him in the last few weeks of his life and was a powerful testimony to the Lord Jesus he gave his life to 37 years before.

Anyone and everyone who came into his room in those final days, staff and visitors alike, were touched and moved deeply and even changed. Staff came into "the most peaceful room in the building"—their words, not mine!

Yes, it was, and still is an emotional rollercoaster, but I was deeply blessed to see my husband's spirit growing stronger and stronger as his physical body faded to nothing.

I thank God that he turned up big time... the Invisible God became a tangible Presence and that was a comfort to all involved with Peter, regardless of any religion or none.

THANK YOU, JESUS; and BLESS YOU Peter for staying the course way beyond our expectations. Job well done; enjoy your Glorious new Home, with those who have gone before you; BUT especially with the Saviour who makes all things possible. Amen, yea and amen.

Suzanne Ross

FOREWORD

Once there was a man called Peter, a preacher who was Chaplain of the United States Senate and pastor of the New York Avenue Presbyterian Church in Washington, D. C., before his early death from a coronary thrombosis. In her book *A Man Called Peter*, his wife Catherine Marshall, recalls the last thing he said to her before the ambulance took him to hospital: "See you in the morning." Later, the hospital called to let her know Peter had died.

This book by Suzanne Ross is also about a man called Peter. Like Catherine Marshall, she is also writing about her husband. Peter Marshall never got to say goodbye to his wife, though his last words were in effect his goodbye, for while she would not see her husband in the morning, she would surely see him again – in the dawn of their new morning together in the Kingdom of God. Why? Because they had both given their lives to their Saviour Jesus; they had faith and hope.

Suzanne Ross had more time to say goodbye to *her* Peter. In fact, they had a prolonged goodbye that extended over a few years. Her Peter did not have a heart attack, but had his life shortened by that debilitating disease that afflicts many – dementia. The prolonged suffering was, in a sense, a blessing, because both had more time to say goodbye, and both had the peace and assurance of ultimately seeing each other again because of their faith in Jesus.

But the prolonged time granted to them also meant coming to terms, day by day, with the gradual loss of Peter's memory, even his identity. Suzanne's confiding style, her heartfelt honesty in her account of the journey through Peter's dementia, makes her book a classic of equal merit to Catherine Marshalls story.

On the one hand you might say the book is about end-of-life care for a dementia patient, in this case a lifelong partner; but far more important is what the author reveals about Providence. The two themes, Dementia and Providence, are woven together, for by virtue of the faith and strong belief in the presence of a loving and extraordinary God, the author is led, step-by-step, through the whole changing experience, right up to Peter's final departure in the care home's end-of-life bed.

She often, in moments of crisis or indecision, uses 'arrow prayers' – prayers shot up to God in moments of urgency. And she always gets an answer. There are a lot of challenges and opportunities for arrow prayers because Peter, as his dementia grows worse and memory loss increases, he will take to wandering in the streets in his slippers, looking for Suzanne even though she has told him she was just popping out to the supermarket. By keeping an open channel to God for prayers, at all times, she has a lifeline at every moment of the day and night.

Prayer and Providence are so woven into the author's life that they become part of the fabric of her life. Decision making at points of need and indecision, like buying a bungalow after seeing the estate agent's photo in the paper, are implemented by prayer; or like the time when an opportunity arises to adopt two Springer Spaniels whose owner is seeking a new home; and of course, the decision whether to put down her beloved Spaniel, Archie, who had terminal cancer; and most importantly, the decision whether to surrender Peter to full-time care in a care home. Prayer works like a synaptic bridge between such moments of decision, allowing you to move on with confidence.

The book is especially valuable for those who are nursing an end-of-life or terminally ill relative, to know what to expect – for the author helps one to anticipate what might happen and what is normal – especially in the last moments of the patient's awareness or consciousness. Her strategy of resting her hand on Peter's hand each time before taking leave of him at the end of a visit is admirable – allowing him to drift off to sleep with a sense of security before she leaves. The reader who might for the first time be living with a terminally ill spouse or parent or child might be able to strengthen the bond between carer and patient in those last moments when the patient's awareness or memory of his or her partner is at a very low ebb, something that might be amplified by medication like morphine. And handling the grief and coming to terms with grief afterwards is so important – and the book will reassure the reader that the acute pain of loss is altogether normal – and here too the author shows that the pain of loss can be ameliorated by handing it all to the Creator, the ultimate Comforter, the *Parakletos*, 'the one beside you'.

If you are new to a dying relative or friend, this book will serve as a forerunner, a guide, so you can know what to expect, and how to face the bitter-sweet pain of saying goodbye.

Charles Muller
MA (Wales), PhD (London), DEd (SA), DLitt (UOFS)

CONTENTS

INTRODUCTION

Who was walking through dementia with Jesus? The naturally obvious answer to that would be – the one who has the dementia. My husband Peter had the dementia – vascular dementia. But we both walked the walk together through it, with Jesus.

Did that really help though? Without a doubt it did. Having three of us walking this walk called 'the long goodbye,' it was as the Bible described in Ecclesiastes 4:12 – the three-corded rope. The Good News translation says that two people can resist an attack that would defeat one person alone. A rope made of three cords is hard to break.

From the beginning I was convinced that Peter and I were walking this walk that would eventually lead to death. It would not defeat us as we knew from many years of experience that Jesus was walking it with us, and He would never forsake us.

CHAPTER 1

NO CURE, BUT…

AFTER THE AMAZING Stephen Hawkins died, a Facebook friend posted a drawing of Stephen walking away from his wheelchair, with computer attached, that had been his home for fifty years. A simple picture but a very powerful one illustrating that at death the spirit leaves the body and is no longer bound by a home, called a wheelchair. I looked intently at it for a while and thought of my husband, that when Peter died on the 5th March 2018 his spirit left his body and his electric end of life bed that had constantly pumped air all around different parts of his body for seven months to keep bed sores at bay. It was as though his spirit walked away unseen, leaving the dementia of thirteen years behind. Its grip on him had only been temporary – it had to let him go!

He is in Glory now, catching up with old friends and family who got there before him, and making new friends he'd never met before. I know he would love to have a chat with some of Jesus' apostles... but most of all I am sure he can't take his eyes off Jesus, the Perfecter of our faith – Who made all things possible for Peter, and for all of us down here, if only we can accept

Him into our lives now as a gift from the Father, as my Peter did many years ago in 1981. Thank you, Lord.

Billy Graham died twelve days before Peter at the age of ninety-nine years. A few years back Billy said: If anyone tells you that Billy Graham has died, tell them – no he hasn't, he has just changed his address and gone to live with his Lord and Saviour, Jesus Christ, in his Eternal home. So as Peter's cremation and celebration service of his life was the beginning of Easter week, I took that on board too and declared: 'Like Billy Graham, Peter didn't die, he just left his body and changed his address to be with his Lord and Saviour, Jesus Christ, in his Eternal Home.'

Still today there is no cure for dementia – it is the most feared disease, is terminal and therefore hopeless. But if you have surrendered your life to Jesus Christ and He has come and taken up residence in your life by the Holy Spirit, then the hopelessness of dementia can be transformed into the wonderful Hope we have to come, in anticipating our Heavenly Home when we leave this earth.

But I must say that I, in my own experience, had to keep trusting in God. That spurred me on in Peter's early days in the dementia nursing home, to ask Him to help me to see positives in every one of the gut-wrenching stages that lay ahead for Peter. And He took me by surprise by promptly starting to answer that prayer. I will leave that to another chapter, and how my heart and my faith began to rise above the circumstances despite everything.

CHAPTER 2

EARLY STAGES

WE GOT OUR FIRST personal computer in the mid-1980's, an Amstrad CPC6128, and we set it up in the living room on a small table behind the settee.

To load anything, you had to buy programmes on cassettes. My favourite was a golf game that took half-an-hour to load from the cassette player. The children were quick learners; I used it mainly for games and Peter didn't really get into it in the early days!

When Ian went to college, Hatfield Polytechnic, to do civil engineering, in 1989, we moved the computer upstairs onto the large and heavy black table in the front bedroom, for their GCE studies. Peter and I got to use it more, and when we chose to install a Sky free sat dish, we not only extended our choice of TV programmes, we were also able to get a broadband package and phone calls – amazing progress at the time. I created an email address and account; Peter did too but wasn't into letter writing as much as I was! For every site we set up on we needed a password to go with the email address – for personal privacy and security.

Eventually Peter and I ventured into the serious business of online banking... so many things to remember – email address, passwords with small letters, capitals and numbers. We were encouraged in these heady days of computing not to use the same password for everything! Peter made notes of these in very small writing in his diary. I got a notebook especially when pass-numbers and three sorts of memorable data were added, like – mother's maiden name, the place you were born, name of your first pet, etc!

Peter was very cautious about banking online – he had worked in a bank for thirty-two years, before, in 1981, he took redundancy and started a new career training to be a nurse. So, he only did his banking when alone in the upstairs room on the computer.

The year 2005, in retrospect, was when I saw signs of what was to come; although I never recognised it as early dementia until a vividly remembered moment in 2008. That was when the penny dropped. The first sign was in 2005, still not recognised as his early signs of dementia: Peter stopped reading in bed. He was a prolific reader of all genres of paperbacks; always had a book by his bed and would every night quietly read well into the early hours. When I occasionally woke up in the small hours, he still had his head stuck in his latest John le Carre or Alistair Maclean. During this year I first noticed he would put his book down before I got to bed. Then the same book was being left on his bedside table for a long time.

One night I asked him: "Peter, you don't seem to be reading in bed anymore." His reply: "Well, I can't remember what was on the page before, so I'm not enjoying it anymore." I simply registered his reply and let it drop.

It was only years later in 2010 when he got a confirmed diagnosis of vascular dementia, that I registered those early signs in 2005. So unaware at the time of what was coming, Peter and I had started to enjoy holidays abroad once the children started opting out of family holidays to do their own thing now as growing up teenagers. Years in Mallorca with Thomson's, and later when Ian had graduated from Hatfield and stayed up there in Hertfordshire, and Christine finished four years at Keele and joined the MV Doulos, Peter and I graduated to Saga holidays in Spain, Malta, Turkey, Cyprus....

In 2006 the children joined us for a family holiday in San Pedro, southern Spain. A great time we had – very special – more to follow. But homeward bound from San Pedro, we collected our car not far from Gatwick airport. Peter was driving. As we approached the big roundabout that would get us down onto the M23 going towards London and the M25 and back home, Peter said: "Which way?" Ian from the back seat simply said: "Straight across, Dad!"

Lo and behold, Peter drove straight across – straight at the roundabout! Ian shrieked: "Left Dad, left!" Peter turned the wheel quickly, all but brushed the curb of the roundabout, and shouted back at Ian: "You told me to go straight ahead!"

There was no damage, no collision, but quite bemused at what had happened, we gave moment by moment instructions and got onto the M25 going in the right direction, thinking no more of it. As I write this years later, that last phrase seems crazy. Dementia was not talked about then; it never crossed our minds.

On our next holiday Peter and I were again flying from Gatwick, and we started using a parking firm a few miles away from the airport. And had a courtesy bus to and from the airport.

To get there and back we went through a small Surrey village, round a roundabout with a very attractive pub on one corner. It was on the way back home after a lovely holiday that we approached this roundabout. No, Peter didn't go straight across! But he did stop suddenly in the middle of the roundabout. I could see a single decker country bus coming up the road from the left about 200 yards away. I said urgently: "Peter, keep going, don't stop in the middle!" He quietly replied: "I'm waiting for that bus to go through." "Pete, you will confuse him, he hasn't got right of way. *You* have – you are already on the roundabout."

But he wouldn't budge and kept his eye on the bus. Fifty yards away the bus slowed down and the driver flashed his lights. "Peter, he's flashed his light at us. He is giving way."

Peter reluctantly pulled forward and waved a hand to thank the bus driver. I resisted any further comment so as not to distract him. I was a bit concerned but I didn't make any connection with the previous roundabout incident. Obviously, I do now.

Later that year, and again in 2007, Ian invited his dad to go and stay with him in his flat in Harpenden. The first time they had a lovely time together and Ian took Pete out for a good meal. And then Ian came back with Peter to stay in Ashford for a break and connect with old school friends. But the second visit to Ian was different. Ian apparently came back in the car with Peter again, but when he saw me, he said: "Never again Mum, I am not going in the car with dad driving ever again."

"Why on earth not, Ian?"

"Remember the Gatwick roundabout last year, mum, when Dad went to go straight across? Well, he did the same thing on the large, busy Luton roundabout!"

Did we think 'dementia' then? No, not at all. Just a bit of old age confusion, not that he seemed that old!

The first incident was over 14 years ago as I write this coming into 2020. But the disease was not talked about very much at all in those days, certainly not up front and often in the press as it is today.

CHAPTER 3

REALISATION – THE PENNY DROPS

SO, when did the penny drop?

I remember the day our neighbour Colin retired as a 'postie' and came home from his leaving party at work. It was well before we suspected Peter as having dementia. In a sense the joke that a friend had shared with Colin at the party and Colin related to me over the fence, turned out to be quite prophetic and a very simple but true definition of dementia. "Sue," he said, "dementia is not forgetting your neighbour's name, it is forgetting that your neighbour IS your neighbour!" Of course, we shared hilarity over the joke, especially as he and his wife had been our neighbours for a number of years and we got on very well with them; we'd never forget who they were, would we... ha!

A couple of years later when Peter was in the system at the hospital for a diagnosis, Peter came up the drive from the front garden and settled in a chair to doze. A nice sunny day, I went outside, saw Colin washing his car and went to natter with him. He stopped, looked at me and hesitated. Then he said that Peter had come out of our back door and walked down the drive towards him. When Colin saw him, he stopped and started to have a conversation with Peter. All he got back was a blank look and a suspicious stare. The conversation was not reciprocated as Peter turned around and went back into the house.

"He clearly didn't know who I was, Sue. I am so sorry."

"Thanks Colin, but as you know, he has been in the system at the hospital for some time, and sooner or later we will get a definite diagnosis. But what comes to mind is the joke about dementia at your retirement party... that still makes me smile, but how very prophetic it has turned out to be; the definition was spot on, and your neighbour doesn't recognize you anymore!"

We both had a giggle which eased the tension of the situation.

For me the penny dropped, heavily into my heart, a couple of years before in 2008 – two years after the first driving 'across' the roundabout incident.

We were coming up to our Ruby Wedding – 40 years of married bliss... not always bliss but it was a good strong marriage, and we had a party prepared to celebrate with old and new friends and neighbours, at the firm's social club where I had a part-time job as a Sensory Panellist, otherwise known as a 'sniffer'. A sunny morning beckoned us to The Broomfields, one of our favourite places to take our Springer Spaniel, Archie, for his daily workout!

We were about to leave when there was a knock on the door, and a couple of local friends for some thirty years had come with a card and a pressie. We had a chat catching up on the latest news. Archie settled back in his bed – he'd been here before! After they left, I picked up the lead, but before we moved Peter looked at me and said: "Who were they?" My heart lurched.

"Janine and Tony," I replied, "You remember them, don't you?"

"No," was his short reply. I looked at him, baffled, but said nothing. He had been chatting away happily with the rest of us – and he didn't remember. That was the moment of realization and the penny dropped. All those early signs were indeed signs of some sort of dementia, I was sure. My heart stayed in my boots as we walked the dog, chatting on and off.

Having gone most of the way around I decided to broach the subject. Peter had a routine appointment with his doctor that afternoon. So, I took a deep breath and said: "You have a doctor's appointment this afternoon; is there anything you are concerned about?"

He replied: "Well yes, I am bit worried about my memory." I felt momentarily relieved – step one. Now for step two. Peter was in many ways a very private person, much more than myself, and had never had me going into a doctor's appointment with him – never needed to… till now. A deep breath, step two: "Would it help then if I came in with you?" No hesitation: "Yes, I think it might."

With this fresh revelation of not knowing two old friends, and his immediate consent to me joining him in the doctors, for the first time in all this my thoughts focused on Jesus. I was now out of my depth as the word 'dementia' kept ringing in my head. I handed an unknown future to our Saviour. Peace settled in my heart.

2.30pm we went to see our favourite doctor – Dr Joe. I was so relieved to be in that room with him and Peter. Who'd have thought this when we woke up this morning? Another arrow prayer. The routine business over, Dr Joe asked if there was anything else. Maybe, I thought, he was a step ahead of us – it was the first time I had gone into a routine appointment with Peter.

"I don't think so," said Pete.

I dived in, "Peter, you said it might be helpful if I came in with you because you were a bit concerned about your memory."

"Oh yes," he replied.

When Dr Joe asked for more Peter couldn't think of anything, so I took over and shared about the incident with our old friends a few hours before. Peter kept quiet. But Dr Joe was on the ball. There were no GP cognitive tests in those days, but I guessed he knew immediately what we were probably dealing with. He said he would get Peter an appointment at the hospital in the next couple of weeks. Having been a GP's receptionist for several years I knew that he was fast-tracking Peter. As we got up and turned to the door, I turned back to shake his hand and mouthed, 'Dementia?' He nodded.

I was both relieved and feeling rather sober; relieved that we were moving quickly on it, sober because there could be a long journey ahead with Peter – a journey totally unfamiliar to me, one where I had no previous experience.

CHAPTER 4

THE LONG GOODBYE

TWO WEEKS after seeing Dr Joe in the summer of 2008 an appointment came for Peter to see a Dr A at the William Harvey Hospital in the Outpatients Dept next door to the Arundel Psychiatric Dept.

She asked loads of questions and took lots of notes. She took her time with Peter and was very patient. Peter answered when he could and looked at me when he couldn't. She arranged for him to have some routine tests and made another appointment to see him.

At the second visit I was hoping she would give some sort of diagnosis. But she didn't. This walk with Peter was becoming a lonely one for me. He was becoming a bit short tempered with me on more and more occasions. If I asked him a question or if I reminded him to take his medication, he would reply sharply. From my point of view all necessary as his 'forgettery' was getting longer. Even what was usually a relaxing fun time, like walking the dog over Hothfield Common, became quite tense at times, as he reacted at some things that didn't even actually exist, but they were my fault. I look back, in retrospect now and realise, that having been a geriatric nurse up until his retirement, he could be more aware of what was going on than I was.

This part of the long goodbye was probably the loneliest time for me. The lady consultant was in no rush to diagnose Peter. More tests were ordered – a CT scan of the head, ex-rays, more blood tests, and a booking to see the consultant in the Respiratory Dept as Peter had suffered sleep apnoea for years. Then followed an appointment with the cognitive specialist, who did a load of numbers and words tests. Now my hopes rose to a decision. To me on this first visit I saw some sort of evidence of dementia…. of cognitive degeneration.

Numbers first – well, Peter was brilliant! The chap gave him a list of six numbers to remember and repeat them back. No problem! Eight numbers – easy! Ten – same result! At last, I was briefly enjoying this and proud of Pete! I did say that Peter had worked in a bank for 32 years and had always most definitely been a numbers person. I was completely opposite and had always been a languages and words person.

Pete was enjoying this – his memory was not struggling. At this point the man decided he would up the stakes. He said he was going to try Peter on 18 numbers, which was one more than the most he had heard anyone recite after him. So, he rolled off the 18 numbers to Peter. I got lost after six! Peter, without hesitation, reeled all back at him, at speed! Absolutely correct. Peter was smiling, really pleased with himself. How he needed that encouragement. It gave me a lesson for the years to come – to always encourage him….and the other folk in the dementia nursing home too.

Then the word games were introduced. First the man told a short story and asked Peter to repeat it. Very slowly he struggled and got some of it. Then the man repeated the story, and started to chat to Peter, passing the time of day. He then asked Peter to repeat the short story. He was completely lost. More word association tests followed. I am a word person and I enjoyed doing them quietly in my head.

It was a different matter for Peter. His memory struggled big time with word tests. And when asked about the original story, it was totally forgotten. Even a little prompting giving a few clues. No recollection at all. I was shocked.

But there was a final test – a very simple test. He just asked Peter to name any words beginning with a given letter in the alphabet, e.g., 'a' in 10 seconds. Peter was clearly out of his depth with this one and got 3 or 4…. a, an, and, about. That took him the 10 seconds. Several attempts and several letters later Peter never managed more than 4 simple words – usually 2 or 3 letters. For me I could do 12 – 15. Now it sank in, in how much his brain WAS beginning to be affected by some type of dementia.

But when this very pleasant and patient man said: "I'll see you again in a year, Peter," I was horrified. I was expecting an instant diagnosis as a result of these tests.

As we went out of the door, I turned back to him and shared what was on my mind and asked, why wait another year? His answer was yes, the word tests were poor, but the numbers were amazing. He would send a report to the senior consultant who asked for the tests. It had been over 3 months since we first saw the consultant and these tests were going to be done again in a year! That's 15 months! I was feeling more and more lonely in my new role of caring for a husband who was becoming more and more dependent on me because of his increasing memory loss. We continued to jump through hoops with appointments every 6 months and tests in between.

Prayer very much became my way of life through all this.

CHAPTER 5

POWER OF ATTORNEY?

WHILST ALL THIS was going on the question of Power of Attorney came up. The first mention was when Peter and I were shopping in town. We were going into BHS to look at suitcases when Peter stopped and said he needed to pop into the bank, and he would come straight back. I said I would stand outside when I had finished in BHS. Well, I seemed to be outside quite a while and no sign of him. I had made sure he had his mobile with him and that it was on. So, I rang it. He answered and said he wouldn't be long. I heard a woman's voice in the background ask if that was his wife on the phone, and when he said yes, she asked to speak to me. She asked where I was. I told her and she asked quietly if I could get up to the bank now as Peter seemed confused and what he was wanting to do was not something she would advise. I said I'd be right there.

I sat down and she was obviously relieved to see me. She carried on with Peter in front of me, explaining to him that what he was wanting to do, in her opinion, was not in his best interest. I listened and then suggested we went home and have a think about it. He looked dubious and a little blank, so she called across to a sub-manager who was passing, talked to him out of Peter's hearing, introduced him to Peter and I and effectively handed it over to him, but stayed with us.

Having been primed by his colleague he suggested to Peter and me, that Peter was a little confused about the best thing to do, and he felt the best at this stage was to do nothing. I nodded and verbally agreed. He suggested that in the case of an elderly customer there are increasing problems with memory that can let us down, and as a bank sub-manager he was so aware of the need for integrity on the bank's part to protect the customer and their finances and would often suggest it was always a good idea to get a Power of Attorney in place, even if it was felt it was not immediately needed. He asked Peter if he had a solicitor. Peter answered that he used to work in the Executor and Trustee Dept of this very bank and did a lot of bank business with elderly customers with the solicitor just a few doors away. The banker suggested a name and got an immediate 'yes' from Peter.

So, the banker now suggested that we popped down there now, and made an appointment. This we did with no problem. Waiting in reception, Peter was pointing out on a board of names of past managers and solicitors, and happily picked out names of men he remembered working with when he worked for the bank up the road.

A young lady solicitor came down and introduced herself, took us into an interview room, chatted to us both briefly and we all agreed to meet again more fully putting POAs in place for both Peter and I because the cost was less to do the two at the same time, and it gave peace of mind to the donors and to the rest of the family. I agreed and told her we had a son and daughter who could be involved. Another meeting was booked.

Discussion with the children followed. I would be Peter's POA, and Christine agreed to be my replacement POA for Peter if I died before him. She also agreed to be my POA. And Ian chose to be named on all document as an interested party in both.

Things had been going swimmingly. Chatting in the bank and in the nearby solicitors was familiar ground for Peter. To the children and I this was new up to now, unknown and unfamiliar ground. But chatting it over at home we all saw the benefits of it, and we had peace of mind about continuing, regardless of the responsibility we were legally going to take on. But Peter was beginning to get a bit anxious about it all, and a tad uncooperative – "Yes, my memory is not as good as it used to be, but wasn't all this unnecessary, and a waste of money?" I knew not to press it at that point. So, I shot up an arrow prayer: "What shall I do, Lord?" Immediately John B came to mind, an old friend married to my 'oldest' friend, Pat. I don't mean she is much older than me. In fact, she is just two days older than me, but we have been friends since about the age of 4 years! Both were now retired from the medical profession; John had been a consultant in geriatric medicine. I rang them and John answered, I started to share about Peter and heard him coming downstairs. So as not to spook Peter, I then turned it over to John to ask me leading questions. He was good, I was just having to answer yes and no to his leading questions. He asked to speak to his old mate Pete, who was pleased to chat to John. They chatted for a while. John was obviously doing most of the talking and presumably asking Peter questions. Peter was slow in responding and I guessed that John knew just what to discuss with Peter, and he was obviously giving Peter advice, because Peter wasn't always agreeing with his friend.

Back to me: "Hi John."

"Sue, it is important that Peter gets a POA into place soon. There is obvious memory loss and significant confusion. If it is left too long, he won't be fit to legally sign the documents, and it will be put in the hands of the Court of Protection, and their concern and responsibility will be solely for Peter. You won't be considered or be able to manage his finances. They will take all that over. Sue, you need to see this is sorted, and have POA in place for Peter very quickly. I have told him. He did listen but doesn't think it is necessary. But he has some sort of dementia, possibly Alzheimer's. But that's not a diagnosis Sue. But for you Sue, I warn you that this is going to be 'the long goodbye'. It will not be easy for you Sue, not for any of you – but you will certainly have some peace of mind once the POA is sorted."

And that is where I first heard the phrase THE LONG GOODBYE, and so it was, and is the reason it is the title of this book.

CHAPTER 6

SORTED

IT WAS GOOD to have chatted with John briefly. It reduced the feeling of being alone and isolated in what I look back on now as the early stages. But for sure those early stages certainly were the most difficult. What I would have done without a solid and wonderful relationship with Jesus I can't imagine.

On our next meeting with the solicitor, Ian came with Peter and me. She had all the paperwork for us to take away and get filled in and went through it all slowly and carefully for all our benefits, but of course especially Peter's. When she asked if we had any questions, Peter immediately chipped in: "I don't see the necessity of all this."

Ian very promptly took the initiative: "Dad, you have spent a large part of your life making sure that Mum will be financially secure because you are a lot older than her. You told me that yourself, Dad. This decision about Power of Attorney is not about dying, Dad, but about living. You have left everything to Mum in your will. But now you have a memory problem which could mean you may lose the ability to make decisions. If that happens, Dad, it will be taken over by the Government and out of Mum's hands, and it will leave her without the security you've worked hard for. Is that what you want to happen, Dad?"

Wow, was I amazed at Ian! His head and his heart worked together, and he couldn't help but open his mouth. I was so proud of him. AND I saw a glint of recognition in Peter's eyes, as Ian finished this beautiful little speech!

"NO," said Peter immediately, "I don't want that to happen."

"Well, Dad, you need to make the decision right now. Any further deterioration with your memory, it will all be out of your hands and Mum's."

Solicitor: "Your son is right, Peter; may I suggest you and your family do two things – a POA for you, and one for your wife too. It is less expensive and gives peace of mind to the whole family. How does that sound to you both, Peter and Sue?"

Peter and Sue – we agreed to go ahead for a POA in place for each of us. More discussion followed in the right direction: I would be Peter's POA, with Christine as mine, and, she would be Peter's replacement POA in the event of my dying before him. So, we took the papers home and Christine also agreed.

Meanwhile Peter had his next appointment with the hospital consultant: still no decision... tests continuing. As she showed us out of her room, she touched my arm.

I turned back and she whispered: "Have you set up POA for Peter?"

"We are getting there," I replied. "We now have the paperwork, but he is still dragging his feet about filling it in and signing it!"

She replied: "You need to get it as soon as possible; his memory is not in a good way." I wanted to say a diagnosis from her would help, but Peter had turned back to us and I was not in the right frame of mind to fire that at her.

So, I enlisted my friend Thelma's help and she came over the next morning and we started filling out all the paperwork. Peter trusted Thelma as a close friend. Time to get signatures on the pages. First page, Peter, as the donor. Thelma very carefully reminding him of the urgency. He signed as the donor. Phew! I signed as his chosen POA to be. Thelma signed as witness to both our signatures.

Now to send paperwork to Chris in Carlisle. That was no problem now that the biggest problem was sorted. I thanked God for my old friend and prayer partner. Papers returned promptly from Carlisle. Chris had signed Dad's and mine and got someone in her Carlisle office to co-sign as a witness of her signatures. With great relief we got all papers back to the solicitor. And they soon came back officially signed, stamped and dated, as now legal documents.

SORTED! And what a long stressful haul that had been – just a small part of the 'long goodbye' John had described and warned us about. We weren't to know we had another eight years ahead of us. But Peace did settle in our hearts having surmounted and resolved this particular marathon.

CHAPTER 7

DEMENTIA NURSE AND DIAGNOSIS

THE POA DOCUMENTS arrived in the post, July 2010, two years after our GP made that tentative diagnosis of dementia and fast-tracked us to the elderly care consultant.

Eight months earlier in January 2010 I was contacted by Rosa – a dementia nurse who wanted to have a meeting with me. I met with Rosa, and she explained that dementia nurses were set up and funded by Dementia UK – a charity set up by the past ITN news reader, John Suchet, who had gone through 'the long goodbye' of dementia with his wife, Bonnie, who started to show signs in her 40's. (*MY BONNIE* is a great book to read about their story, written by John himself. As I write now, John Suchet is a well-known presenter on the radio programme Classic FM.)

When I met Rosa, she explained that she was a qualified nurse in the first group trained with funds from Dementia UK, to care for the carers of dementia sufferers. So, in effect, I had a dementia nurse looking out for my well-being, as the carer of a dementia sufferer. Brilliant idea – well done, John Suchet, and thank you.

But the very person who appointed Rosa, and who was Rosa's boss, was Peter's consultant, who seemed very reluctant to give him a diagnosis.

Rosa was a blessing. We met regularly and it was good to talk through the issues with someone outside of family and friends, who was not emotionally involved with it all. After meeting for several months, she asked to meet me at our home so that she could meet with Peter and get an overall feeling of where we were, in situ.

She soon saw that Peter was more advanced than she had realised, so she talked to me about Attendance Allowance, and Carer's Allowance. The latter was for someone totally caring for someone in their own home, e.g., a husband or wife looking after their spouse. It was means tested and was anyway preceded by Attendance Allowance, which was not means tested and was awarded to improve or help with quality of life for both sufferer and carer. And that fitted the bill for Peter and me. I remarked that Peter had still not been diagnosed by her boss who had appointed Rosa to be my dementia nurse. She said she would have a word with Peter's consultant about that, because he couldn't get Attendance Allowance until he has an official diagnosis.

An appointment arrived within a week, and the following week we were in the consultant's office. She gave me a letter of confirmation that she was diagnosing Peter as suffering from vascular dementia but was not sure he didn't have a combination of two types of dementia. As we talked, she still seemed to be hedging her bets. So, I asked her why she hadn't given a diagnosis months earlier when she had appointed Rosa as my dementia nurse, to support me in my caring for Peter. Her answer was brief: "Because we don't like to put a label on people too soon." I said that I would very much have appreciated an earlier diagnosis, because it had been a long and lonely path of two years with Peter, since 2008, when his GP had fast tracked an appointment for Peter with her. Both Dr Joe and I had agreed that day that we felt it was some form of dementia.

Of course, things have changed since then. Now GPs are encouraged to use cognitive tests to diagnose dementia quickly. The initial incentive to move the process along was, I believe, a £55 fee. That I believe was later discontinued, in about 2014. It was questioned ethically, and the momentum to early diagnosis was now general practice anyway.

But for Peter, POA was in place and a diagnosis had been established. All necessary steps had been taken along the way, on this road, this very uneven road of this 'long goodbye' of dementia. A lot more of a never-before travelled journey lay ahead. Why people go to fortune tellers to have their future foretold I just don't know.

I had no idea what lay ahead except that with no cure, this was a terminal disease. How much gratitude I felt then, and increasingly at each stage, that I had a Heavenly Father covering me – and indeed all of us in the family. And HE was the only one who knew the end from the beginning. He was, unknown to me in those early stages, going to do a major work in my life, teaching me how to take a day at a time, always leaving tomorrow in His hands.

CHAPTER 8

NORMAL LIFE CONTINUES...
SORT OF!

WITHIN a couple of months of Peter's diagnosis and us setting up the POAs, I had my first book published – *An Ordinary Person with An Extraordinary God*.

I had been brought up churched as a child by my mum in South Wales, christened and confirmed in a high Anglo Catholic church in Newport. I certainly always believed that God existed, and I often went to church alone at 8am on a Sunday morning.

But though I believed in God, I had no idea there was more until one night at the age of thirty I had an encounter with God that felt like time stopped and it lasted for ever, but it was about twenty minutes, because I heard the evening news ending on the telly downstairs. I knew for certain that I had met with God; he moved me to pray non-stop for my dad in Cornwall, who'd always claimed to be an atheist, which annoyed Mum. Just as suddenly as I started to pray, I stopped. And I was bathed in a wonderful warmth and light. I also knew for certain that 300 miles away my dad had just died and he was safe with God.

That story can be read in that first book in the chapter – FIRST ENCOUNTER WITH THE LIVING GOD. That was April 13th, 1976. And my Dad DID die at 9.20pm on that night.

Eighteen months later, God had never let go of me from that moment and I came to a point when I couldn't and didn't want to hold out any longer, and I surrendered my life to Jesus Christ, was born again, and two days later I had a Pentecostal experience, being filled with the Holy Spirit and praying out in a new language.

That changed my life forever. I'd had religion but I discovered religion does not produce salvation. Relationship does. Salvation comes when one comes into a relationship with Jesus Christ, by being born spiritually. Jesus Himself insisted: "Very truly I tell you, no one can enter the Kingdom of Heaven unless they are born of water and the Spirit." John 3:3. That means that to be assured of Eternal Life, it is essential to be born twice – physically and spiritually.

Peter kept his own counsel but watched my life change after I had met with Jesus. He followed and gave his life to Jesus in 1981 whilst riding his Honda 50 motorbike going to work. He said later: "I was riding up Hythe Road when I decided to ask Jesus into my life. The heat that went through my body from head to foot totally surprised me and nearly threw me off my bike. So, I stopped and stood still for a while until I felt in a fit state to continue!"

On November 26th, 1995, Peter and I were baptised in the sea in Mallorca. We were united in Christ. Little did we know how the strength of being united in marriage and united in Christ would work for us in the worst of scenarios – Peter, once diagnosed with vascular dementia, had a terminal disease. No hope of surviving it physically… no treatment or cure. It would end sooner or later in his death. But we did have hope – we both shared in the Eternal Hope, that would never let us down.

So, I wrote my story between 2006-2008, and got it published with Diadem Books in 2010.

By then I was very much Peter's carer. I had given up my job as a 'sniffer' at Givaudan, and left hospital chaplaincy after 21 years; and gave up church leadership and associated commitments. I aimed to help him live life to the full at every stage. We went Sainsbury's shopping together and Peter's mobility in later days was greatly helped by him pushing the trolley! We continued to take Archie, our Springer Spaniel, daily over Hothfield Common. And we continued with Saga holidays abroad – Turkey, Cyprus, Malta, Spain, Ibiza, the Canary Islands. Saga were brilliant – very sensitive to Peter and my responsibility for him. The Saga reps were always so helpful, often going the extra mile to make sure we had a good holiday, and I had a bit of a rest too.

CHAPTER 9

RESPITE CARE

IN **2011**, a year after the official diagnosis, Rosa, my dementia carer nurse, advised me to have a break from caring for Peter – respite care for him in a dementia care facility.

I struggled with her suggestion – a rush of mixed emotions gathered inside of me – guilt, denial, a fleeting sense of relief closed by: 'I am coping,' words to myself and to Rosa.

She gently insisted that I would be fitter to look after him at home longer if I took respite breaks with Peter in the safe environment of a dementia care unit or care home. In the end I took charge of the situation by suggesting a week in early December so that I could be free to do all the Christmas shopping and preparations, without my responsibility for Peter.

It was arranged for him to five days in West View Hospital, Tenterden – an NHS hospital with a small dementia unit. Peter seemed compliant with the idea, but his reactions to anything could be erratic. So, a good friend, Roger, agreed to take us both over in his car rather than me driving Peter on my own. This was a relief because recently Peter had tried twice to get out of the car when I was driving. Once he succeeded; I was at traffic lights changing and had to move, and I had to drive around the town centre ring road three times, looking for him, until I saw him walking off the ring road down Mace Lane, quite a distance from home but in the right direction!! I couldn't help but smile at that and stopped and picked him up.

We got to West View – no one at reception, so we made our way down the only corridor. This was indeed a small unit, and I led the way to what seemed to be a lounge at the end. A tall teddy bear of a nurse with a friendly face came toward us. I stepped ahead of Peter and Roger to introduce myself and Peter – not needed! The nurse carried on straight past me, thrust his big hand out, took Peter's firmly in his and shook it firmly: "Peter Ross, we have been looking forward to meeting you, and having you to stay for a little break!"

Peter smiled back spontaneously, and not looking back he went confidently with 'nurse' down to meet the others! Roger and I were left to unpack Peter's bags and put his clothes away, and familiar ornaments where he would see them – to make him feel at home. John, the nurse, had already done that! He brought Peter back up to his room and they both waved us cheerfully goodbye.

Five days later we went back to collect Peter, wondering how he had got on. I was well rested and had managed to get a lot of Christmas preparation done and dusted!

"I wonder if Peter has been all right in here?" I muttered to Roger. It was teatime and we were led down to the lounge. What a lovely lay out – very home from home! Four old ladies were playing cards and they all greeted us. Peter was sitting in front of the 'bar' at the far end.... non-alcoholic that is, but it looked like a bar, where folk could get cool drinks or coffee, and snacks. The lady nurse with us called: "Peter, Sue's here to collect you; come and meet her." He waved, and got up, came over and gave me a hug. He seemed very relaxed and happy and comfortable in himself in this place.

Nurse took his hand and said: "It's lovely, Peter, to have met you and have you with us for a while." He leaned forward and gave her a smacker of a kiss on the cheek! Two other staff, washing up on the other side of the room, called out: "What about us, Peter!" He went over to both of them and another nurse just walking in and gave them all a kiss! I thought: 'Gosh, this is the happiest I have seen him for ages. If in the future this could be his permanent home I wouldn't mind the drive over here to visit him, to see him so content and flourishing.

Sadly, that was not to be. For when it eventually became necessary to transfer Peter to a permanent home, West View was out of bounds. It was an NHS unit – for respite it took anyone, but for permanent care it took only Tenterden people, folk with no finances to cover them in private care. It was obvious that in the years since the then government closed all psychiatric hospitals and brought the care of the mentally ill into the

36

community that the numbers of private care homes, including dementia nursing homes, had mushroomed in the community.

The next respite care I asked for Peter was the next summer, when my friend Thelma and I were on our first trip to Ffald-y-Brenin – a retreat and prayer centre in the wilds of West Wales. West View had no spaces, and we were directed to a new build BUPA dementia care and nursing home, about five minutes' drive from home. So, Peter's second respite spell was in Warren Lodge. And again, I was relieved he was safe, and I could have a break in dear old Wales, land of my birth!

Another short pre-Christmas break followed so that I could spend time getting ready for the festive season. I could see that Peter wasn't as content here as in West View. That had been about a nine-bed unit, whereas Warren Lodge had something in the region of sixty-five rooms, on two floors. I suppose it was less homely and more institutionalised. But for now, it was for short breaks only and he was fine.

CHAPTER 10

THE BIG CROSSROADS

THE YEAR 2012 was the year when Peter started to have increased episodes of chest infections. Dr Joe started adding steroids to reinforce the antibiotics and keep at bay what was becoming the inevitable next chest infection. Instead of just a few days in between, the steroids stretched the gap to two weeks between infections. And as it is for all of us in our climate, it was the winter months that were the worst for Peter.

After Christmas 2012 Joe suggested I took Peter away for a longer break to warmer climes. He knew we had been exploring the Canaries for several years, usually in January or February. It had a lovely warm and gentle climate all the year around because of the Atlantic Drift. These islands had, despite being off the Sahara coast of Africa, temperatures affected by the breeze off the Atlantic. So, January averaged 21C, and high summer temperatures averaged 28C – a gentle 7C difference between the coolest and warmest seasons.

Peter and I had been several times to Tenerife and loved it. Now Joe was suggesting we took a month's winter holiday in the Canaries. I quickly gave Saga a ring and in minutes had booked four weeks, early February to early March 2013 in Gran Canaria. Both the children jumped at the idea of an opportunity to be involved. Chris was still in Carlisle working for OM. So having booked four weeks for Peter and me from Gatwick, then also I booked the first ten days for Chris to join us, flying from Manchester; and Ian was booked in for the last two weeks.

What a brilliant holiday that turned out to be! I looked up the hotel on its own website and saw that they had two-bedroomed bungalows beside the pool amongst the trees. I wondered…

Memories of visiting my publisher in Scotland, a few years before, flashed back vividly one memory I didn't want to repeat. As guests we were given our host's double bed for the night. I awoke suddenly to Peter shouting about the soldiers coming on horses and both his hands were gripping my very arthritic knee as though he was fighting off an enemy, more like strangling one, except it was my knee!

It took some time shouting and thumping him for him to let go. I switched on the light and looked at my red and swollen knee.

"Peter, what were you doing? Were you dreaming about being attacked? I am not the enemy, you were strangling my knee, it could have been my neck."

As he fully woke up, he was horrified at what he had done, and we were both shaking with shock. Dawn was coming up and as we calmed down, I drew the curtains back to let the light in as the sun rose, so that both of us could see where we were. I decided it would be safer not to sleep in the same bed or even the same room again.

So, when I saw 'two-bedroomed bungalows' available, I rang Saga and told them, and asked them to ring the hotel and explain our situation and confirm that I was willing to pay the extra. No problem – done and dusted! It worked out as £175 per week extra for each of us, and it provided Peter and I with a great quality holiday with no dementia linked problems. Chris was booked in a single room for 10 days with us, then Peter and I had four days for just the two of us, before Ian arrived for the fortnight. The next bonus we discovered was they had a system of reserved sunbeds – they gave customers at check-in a card with their names and arrival and departure dates. There were plenty of sunbeds all over the grounds, in the sun, or even on grassy slopes under trees. When you go to hotels where there aren't enough sunbeds for everyone, you give up trying and have a swim and go back to your balcony! This hotels arrangement put Quality with a capitol Q into our holiday here for a month. The Manager was checking us in that day, so I told him our daughter was coming in on the next flight from Manchester, and could she have a room in the hotel where she could see our bungalow. "That's Christine Ross," he said without hesitation. I nodded. "No problem," he smiled, "It's all in hand!"

Peter and I went to find our bungalow, with our own little garden with sunbeds. We took our sunbed tickets and hung them on two together opposite our bungalow, with partial tree shade. Brilliant! I felt blessed! In the bungalow we had four rooms – bathroom, two bedrooms, and a living room with a kitchen area. Great!

But the best surprise of that day was when Chris turned up at our bungalow having asked directions. When I asked her, pointing up to the main building overlooking the pool, which room was hers, she just smiled. It dawned on me what the manager meant when he said in response to my request that Chris had a room overlooking the pool so she could see our bungalow: "It's all in hand, Mrs Ross."

"Chris, you're not in a bungalow as well, are you?" She giggled: "Yeh!" and pointed back up the path to the bungalow three doors away!

I went to reception and the manager was on duty there and asked if everything was all right. I said: "You have put our daughter in a bungalow near to us?" He nodded and smiled: "No charge – that's on the house, Mrs Ross!"

Chris had ten days with us and then had to get back to work in the UK. We'd had the best of times together.

Peter and I now had four days, just the two of us, before Ian arrived from Gatwick for the second two weeks with us. I decided, wisely I felt, not to let the blood rush to my head and chance my luck or cheek with the manager again to ask him if Ian could be in a room overlooking the pool so he could see Dad and me. Anyway, there didn't seem to be any bungalows vacant. Even the one

Christine had been in was quickly cleaned and bottles of water had been left on the little windowsill for the next occupants. I was told by the staff member checking it that there was a German couple coming in.

Ian arrived after an uneventful flight – knowing him, he probably slept all the way! He came looking for us – reception had told him where Peter and I were. Greetings and hugs, and then the obvious question: "Which room are you in? Can you see us from there?"

He grinned and said: "I'm not in a room, Mum!" still grinning.

"You're not in a bungalow, are you?" He nodded still grinning! He led the way back up the path and guess what? Instead of putting the yet faceless Germans in the one that Chris had vacated, they had relocated them and kept Chris' one vacant until Ian arrived!

We were all obviously delighted. We had a great month's holiday, Peter and I, the best hotel we'd been in, super Saga rep, great food, and wonderful hotel manager. He put both the children in the bungalows at no extra charge.

A memorable family holiday. And we weren't to know that would be our last holiday as a family. Only one Person knew ahead of us, and I thank and praise God from the bottom of my heart for the blessings of our time together over that month February to March 2013.

That holiday was to be the big crossroads in all our lives. For we weren't to know that was to be the last time Peter would be able to go away on holiday again. A month later he developed a lump in his lower leg and a swollen foot. A DVT was diagnosed and for six months I was to give him injections in his stomach.

CHAPTER 11

HORIZONS ARE REDUCED

A **MONTH LATER** we were into April, and something happened that set the compass for the future, and it was a sound I never want to hear again. I was upstairs in the spare bedroom on the computer whilst Peter was watching telly. I came out of the room to go into the bathroom. I glanced downstairs and saw the top of Peter's head. He was carrying a tray of two cups with hot water in them, the sugar bowl and milk and tea bags. I had noticed recently that he was getting confused about making a cup of tea, and he was used to bringing me a cuppa if I was working upstairs. Usually, he would shout up to me: "Would you like a cuppa Sue?" Invariably I would shout back: "Yes, I will be down in a sec!" And I would go down and we would sit on the settee drinking tea together, watching telly.

He didn't call up this time and I was shocked to see him carrying a tray of 'ingredients' up the stairs. I was going into the loo; he hadn't seen or heard me, and I decided to resist the temptation to tell him to be careful, so as not to distract him. I sat on the throne and then heard him fall – bumping all the way down the stairs backwards and the breaking of china. I was stuck for a few moments where

I was, and I felt sick. I never want to hear that sound ever again. I called out his name desperately several times, as I got up. NO answer. My heart was in my boots and thumping; the silence was deafening, and my immediate thought was a broken neck I shouted again as I got out onto the landing. I heard a moaning sound.

A sense of relief returned to a small degree. He continued to groan as I went down the stairs. There was tea and sugar all over the place and over him – sticky and messed up in his clothes and hair. He didn't seem to be in pain and asked for help to get up. He was between the settee and reclining chair, so we had some leverage and I managed to help him to sit on the end of the settee. Then he wanted the toilet. How fortunate we had built a small bedroom en-suite extension out into the back garden from the dining room. I helped him to walk very slowly there. He still didn't seem to be in pain, but he was struggling a bit, so I sat him on the bed to give him a break, and then helped him into the loo just three feet away.

Then he sat down on the bed again to get his breath back. Did he want to lie down? No. But I noticed he was starting to shiver even though he was fully dressed. So I rushed upstairs to get his dressing gown and helped him on with it. He continued to shiver, but still answered 'no' when I asked him again if he was in any pain anywhere. I suspected then that he was going into shock. So, I rang 999 and asked for an ambulance.

They arrived in about ten minutes, did all the basic checks on him – no obvious fractures but he was definitely going into shock, so they took him in to the local hospital, and I followed by car. I sat with him for the next few hours, wide awake, with the adrenaline pumping through me!

For Peter dementia and hospital beds didn't go well together, as was my experience several times during this long goodbye that is dementia. He wouldn't keep still – they had a real job on their hands. As they got on with the regular necessary checks, blood tests, x-rays, CT scans, Peter fidgeted and tried to get out of bed or off the trolley a number of times. The nurse put in charge of him was a saint to look after him as she did!

I started to flag at about 5am – I'd used up all my available adrenalin! At 5.30am the duty consultant came in with CT scans that had been taken and put then on the screen and switched the light on. I joined him and asked him to explain them to me, which he did. Peter had fractured his pelvis on both left and right sides. Fortunately, they were simple fractures, no surgery required or advised. He needed to be admitted and would be on bed rest until it healed. My silent thought: 'My goodness, you may have to put him in a strait jacket!!' But I followed that quickly with a silent prayer: 'Into Your hands Lord – his healing is in your hands.'

I left Peter, being distracted by a nurse, in A&E waiting to be moved up to the surgical ward. Peace settled in my heart as I drove home. The sense of responsibility dropped away. He was in a safe place. I got home and sat down for breakfast at 6.45am. Sleep evaded me. So I then tidied and cleaned up the remains of his fall – sticky patches of tea and sugar and water down the stairs and over the living room floor. And then I sat down quietly with Jesus and thanked Him that it wasn't much more serious and prayed for Peter's speedy healing and recovery; and strength for me to go with Peter through the next stage of this cruel disease. I texted both the children about the situation, (Ian lived in Harpenden, and Christine in Carlisle); then I returned to the hospital at about 10am.

A few weeks later Tayo (name changed), the Social Services manager in the hospital, gave me a call and asked if we could meet to discuss future plans for Peter. I arranged to meet her the next afternoon on the ward. Sitting at a small desk across the ward from Peter, I met a lovely, smiling Nigerian Lady. I was taken by surprise because when she had given me her name, her surname was Dutch! She called my name, and I went over and mentioned her name, and she laughed and said she was Nigerian, married to a Dutchman. We were getting on very well and I was relieved to have her in charge of the next stage of Peter's recovery.

After about five minutes she stopped and looked intently at me: "You are a born-again Christian, aren't you Sue?" Joy hit me – "Yes, and you are too?" She nodded. We were well away then – only just met but, as the saying goes, we were 'singing from the same hymn sheet!'

Down to business – she discussed with me about getting Peter out of hospital into a care unit for about two weeks, funded by the NHS, where a nurse/physiotherapist would work with him for his optimum physical recovery, to get him back on his feet. I agreed after asking several probably obvious questions, but of course this was new ground to me. Peter, in the bed opposite, had by now dozed off. Tayo looked back to me and said: "Let's pray for him and ask God to heal him." I readily agreed, so we did just that, gave each other a hug, and she left. I had had time with Peter, before the meeting, and now he was sleeping soundly, so I grabbed my coat off the chair beside his bed, and quietly left and went home, very thoughtful and at peace.

I went in to visit him the next day. There was a walking aid by his bed. Nurse came to speak to me. Apparently after I had left the previous afternoon, Peter woke up, got out of bed and walked to the loo. I gaped in amazement!

"He's been a real problem," she said. "We tell him to call us if he wants to go to the bathroom, but he just gets up and goes there himself… AND he locks the door on the inside; and now he has started wandering into other bays as well. He won't rest, so we have given him a walker to keep him steady and safe, but he just won't use it!"

The smile I was holding onto cracked open as she turned away and went on with her work. "Wow, Lord, it only this time yesterday that Tayo suggested we pray for

Peter's healing! It seems you have healed his fractured pelvis and now he's a big problem for the staff because he won't stop going walkabout!" I drove home with this silly grin on my face! I left a message for Tayo on her phone, so that that she could rejoice with me, which of course she did.

When I went in the next day, I met her coming out from behind the curtains around Peter's bed. We had a big hug, but there was more to share. She was obviously excited about something else. She told me that the next day there was to be a big team meeting to decide about Peter. It looked as though there was a strong general feeling that he needed to go into permanent care. I could understand that – he now was the advanced dementia patient who was wandering everywhere, and a hospital ward is not the safest of places for the customer, or other patients. Yes, it seemed God had healed his physical fractures, but that brought things to a head and conference time! So, what was it that she was excited about? She related a conversation she had just had with Peter. She asked him if he was prepared to go into a permanent care home.

His answer: "Well, I don't want to, but if my wife Sue can't cope with looking after me, then I will."

"What about the dangers in going home, Peter?"

"What dangers?"

"Well, you are in hospital because you fell backwards down your stairs at home and fractured your pelvis. Obviously, the stairs are a danger for you."

Peter: "What is the point of worrying about something that might never happen. I will sleep in my own bed and be very careful on the stairs!"

Now was the time for my mouth to drop open in amazement, just as I had seen hers as she came from behind his curtain.

"Sue," she said, "I was amazed. His dementia is quite particularly advanced, yet he spoke clearly, logically, and made his wishes clear. I will recommend that he has two weeks in a local home, with physiotherapy, with a view to going home. I cannot, after hearing how he spoke and what he said, recommend a permanent care home. What I will do tomorrow, before the meeting, is take the senior staff nurse on his ward to see him with me and again I will ask him the same question."

"Ok Tayo, I am amazed too. He is walking around apparently healed after we prayed for him, and now he is talking so logically he wouldn't seem to have dementia. If he gives you the same answer tomorrow, I will vote to take him home!

The next day Chris and I arrived a little early for the meeting. Peter's curtains were closed. After a few minutes out came Tayo and the staff nurse and they both confirmed he had answered the same question in the same way.

We all went into the meeting – quite a comprehensive bunch – ward staff, doctor, care assistant, psychiatrist, social services, and family, i.e. Chris and me. And a comprehensive discussion took place too.

Two suggestions were made. The first was that Peter would go into a local care home where a physiotherapist would work with him to build up his physical strength and mobility, and then a more permanent assessment on his future would be made. The second suggestion was that he went immediately into a dementia care home. That suggestion was immediately rejected by Tayo, Chris and me. We shared briefly the conversation that Tayo had with Peter and only minutes before this meeting with the staff nurse. But I certainly went along with the suggestion that Peter goes into a local care home for two weeks' assessment and physiotherapy. If he was to come back home again I obviously was aware that he was unstable on his feet. So that was my choice, and the decision was made. I did suggest Ashminster House, the nearest dementia care home virtually at the top of our road. There was a delay in getting him in any such unit at that time, as there was no vacancy in any unit.

Meanwhile Peter could be discharged home in my care with a care package in place to help him and support me as his main care support. I would continue with the DVT injections. A care firm was contacted, and Caroline arrived to meet Peter. It was decided that the best help for my benefit, because of my arthritis, was that she came first thing, about 8am each day, get Peter up, help him to wash, shave and get dressed, and then get him down the stairs, and I would sit down to breakfast with him.

Also, to make him as safe as possible at home, the hospital team would immediately arrange a lifeline package to be in place – an emergency buzzer for his wrist and one around his neck with its own emergency phone system connected to our phone line, and a key safe on an outside wall so that in an emergency the ambulance men could let themselves in. That was promptly up and running within 24 hours, with Shepway Lifeline. All we had to wait for now was the vacancy in a local care home for Peter to have a two-week stay for physiotherapy and assessment.

CHAPTER 12

A BUMPY ROAD AHEAD

PETER wasn't the easiest of customers or, to put it another way – dementia is so unpredictable. Sometimes he cooperated with Caroline and at others he was as awkward as he could be. She was very experienced and took it all in her stride, and I learned a lot just from observing her!

About a week later we heard there was a room for him in Ashminster House for him, for the two-week stay of assessment and physiotherapy. We were delighted – that was just at the top of our road and opposite both our church and doctor's surgery. We were to take him in the evening of the 9th May 2013. When we arrived, there was just evening staff on duty and Peter was in a room on the ground floor. A very young Spanish care assistant led us to Peter's room. I must admit that I was already feeling a little uneasy – first that he was on the ground floor not far from the front door – might he try to escape if he knew! Also, I was expecting him to be upstairs where the dementia unit was; and he was admitted in the evening when there was only a small number of staff. Perhaps I was overreacting. But no, for the young and seemingly inexperienced carer was talking to Peter in an inappropriate manner, treating him in a too familiar and condescending way, telling him off for being like a naughty boy when he had only spoken to me and Chris querying where he was and why. So, her unprofessional teenager style of butting in was certainly getting him aggravated. I felt she was being rude to him. I thanked her and she left. I chatted to Peter briefly about my birthday the next day and we would come in to see him and he could help me open my presents and cards. We left him to settle down and promised to be in the next day after lunch with a cake and candles for us to share. He seemed happy enough with that, and we left.

Next morning, 10th May 2013, my 66th birthday! My friends Barbara and Sylvia treated me to a cream tea at Dobbies. I drove back via the motorway to drop Sylvia off on the Highfield estate. Barbara was next, not far from mine. My mobile rang twice as I was driving on. So I stopped and picked up a voicemail from Ashminster House, to go there as soon as possible. 'Oh, gosh, what has Peter been up to!' I wondered. I dropped Barbara off and went straight to the care home.

Lots of staff there during the day, including the manager. They were obviously trying to keep Peter distracted in the entrance hall, one of them guarding the front door. The manager beckoned me to her office. She had apparently called for an ambulance, and the police. Peter had got up from the lunch table and said he was going home. Two members of staff had tried to stop him before he got to the front door. The first one he twisted her wrist, the second had her finger bent right back.

Peter went for the front door and within seconds had it open and was on his way out! Another member of staff met him on the pavement and persuaded him to come and have a cup of tea with him, and wait for Sue, his wife, who was on her way. Peter weighed all that up and went back inside with him.

I arrived and found him sitting on an easy chair, quite agitated. They brought me a cup of tea and he asked for one too. And he settled down. In about ten minutes a paramedic arrived on his motor bike. He spoke to the manager, and then to me. He had cancelled the police, as totally inappropriate, and the ambulance was being kept on hold. I relaxed… at last some common sense. Looking back in retrospect and years more experience of dementia and the internal working of a dementia care home under my belt, I knew my instincts at the time were right. The way this home was dealing with this dementia situation displayed a lot of inexperience and a lack of appropriate training and panic. John, the paramedic, drew a chair up and sat down the other side of Peter and started chatting quietly with him. Peter calmed down and was obviously willing to chat with this 'nice' man! John then made, as a precaution, the decision to get the ambulance to take Peter and I to A&E. They would be waiting for him and would assess him and hopefully clear him to go home.

Which is what happened; by the end of the day Peter and I were back home in Cradlebridge. So that was a memorable birthday for all the wrong reasons!

Well, in one day that was the speedy end of the two weeks' physio and assessment idea! The carer continued to come in every morning, and that was a great help for me. Next was the offer of a trial for Peter at Ashford Carer's Day Centre in South Ashford; if it went well, they would increase the number of days. He was to be picked up after breakfast and brought home at 3pm. I got him ready the first day – he was a bit dubious about going – it was something new for both of us to get used to, but more so for him. The minibus arrived, and I answered the door bell. Two friendly guys about sixty spoke to me; they knew it was Peter's first time and that he had dementia. I called: "Peter, there's somebody to see you, really looking forward to meeting you!" Peter came to the door and Bill, and the driver, Mick, put out their hands to greet Peter, and started chatting to him. They obviously had the knack, were experienced in this, and Peter took Bill's offered arm and relaxed as Mick went ahead to open the door; and Peter, prompted by Bill, turned and waved to me, got into the transport and turned and waved at me from the window as they drove off, with other customers waving to me too.

I had given up my job at Givaudan as a 'sniffer', and also over twenty years working on the chaplaincy team at the William Harvey Hospital. I started using the computer more and more because as Peter's dementia progressed, he got increasingly anxious if I left him in the house alone. So, I took him to Sainsbury's to do the weekly shop with me. That didn't turn out to be the burden I thought it might be… in fact, it was a blessing!

Peter was becoming more and more of a faller; he asked to push the trolley whilst I did the shopping and that kept him steady on his feet, and me free to browse down the aisles.

The first day he went to the day centre, 10am to 3pm, I felt like a woman liberated. Peter was safe, and I was free from concern for him. A weight had dropped off me and I floated on air! It so took me by surprise that tears dripped down my face, and I thanked God for the blessings of these days. Although I got used to it after a few weeks, I always appreciated the opportunity of free time from caring!

CHAPTER 13

FFALD Y BRENIN

MY DEMENTIA CARE NURSE kept pestering me to take another respite care break. I had had the short one for Christmas shopping 2012. I had had my last holiday with Peter that lovely month in Gran Canaria, February/March 2013. After the DVT in April 2013 another door was closed on our life together.

At that time someone gave me a book about Ffald y Brenin, a Christian Retreat Centre and House of Prayer right out in the wilds of West Wales between Fishguard and St David's and between mountains and valleys. I couldn't put the book down till I had read the last page. I wondered, 'What a place for a respite break!' And so to restore my batteries, body, soul and spirit, I checked it out online and there at the end of June was a five-day, Monday to Friday personal retreat. Oh, I prayed; then I rang my prayer partner Thelma, and shared with her about it. She had already heard about it and would check with work and get back to me. Yes, it's a go, if they have spaces! I immediately rang Ffald y Brenin, and yes, they had just the room for us. I booked immediately, and they would send me confirmation. What about Peter? We obviously by now were looking for a permanent dementia care home in the not-too-distant future. We knew that the Tenderden unit he had a few happy days in was not able to take him on a permanent basis because he was financially viable to pay for his own care, and the Tenderden unit was for permanent local NHS patients. We had been discussing this with the local medics and my Dementia nurse, and they suggested that we try for Pete's next respite break Warren Lodge, in Ashford, a new place that had been open for about four years. So that's what we did, and we booked Pete in there for that week in June, so it covered our break in Ffald y Brenin and our travelling time. What a blessed time that was – out in the middle of nowhere in the beautiful West Wales, the clean air that has a fragrance of its own, and no mobile phone signal! The freedom to be me with Jesus. The sense of His Presence tangible – never been in a place like this before.

After a pre-lunch worship time I came away with a growing sense of sadness I couldn't explain. Back in our room preparing lunch I tried to explain to Thelma. She looked at me and said: "You need some time alone with Jesus." I certainly knew that. It had started to rain, and everyone knows the rain in Wales is wetter than anywhere else! I looked out of one of our room windows and past the tree-covered path down the slope from the building and saw clearly again the larger-than-life solid wooden cross on the edge of the property. There was nobody down there, the rain was coming down fast and all those on retreat would be having their lunch. Thelma was quiet beside me, and I felt Jesus whisper: "Come away Sue, come away with me."

I immediately got up, put my kagool on, and told Thelma where I was going. As I walked down the path away from the building, and down through the arbour of trees I could hear the light rain on the trees. A gate at the end opened into a quiet space with immediately a seat for those who wanted time alone to pray and contemplate the cross about fifteen yards away on a bit of a rocky outcrop. I kept going and carefully got myself right up to the cross with a view of the narrow road we had come on a long way down in the valley. All I wanted to do was wrap my arms around this rough wooden cross. My experience was of a tremendous power in that place, and an overwhelming Peace was mine, and I closed my eyes, and the wind was blowing, and the rain was lashing down by now; I had come away as invited by Jesus and He had His arms around me, holding me tight, keeping me safe.

He showed me all that I needed to know at that time. I was grieving, over Peter. In all the business of caring and being responsible for him, I never had time for my own thoughts and tears. I had wrapped my arms around that cross, and He held me, and time stood still, the rain lashed down, symbolising how many tears I had never shed. Eventually I let go of that piece of wood but knowing that Jesus was still holding me in His arms all the way back to my room.

And from that point in time, that one beautiful experience of my wonderful Lord and Saviour, He never let me go. Jesus held me through all the ensuing stages of the long goodbye of dementia, until Peter's last breath, and after.

CHAPTER 14

ON THE MOVE

BACK HOME from Ffald y Brenin, rested, restored, and blessed, I went to pick Peter up from his little break in Warren Lodge. Yes, he had asked for me a few times but had enjoyed the music and activities and eaten well. When he needed fulltime care, they would be happy to have him as a resident. I was now very confident that God had the timing of these issues in hand, and I would know the right time for all future decisions.

So back to the routine we had both left for a week – the carer coming in each morning to help get Peter up, and his days at the day centre continued.

A couple of weeks after returning from Ffald y Brenin, I was sitting quietly flicking through the pages of the *Kentish Express*, for the Ashford area, having as usual picked up a weekly copy when shopping in Sainsbury's. I reached the properties for sale pages flitting through the pictures, when something caught my eye, and my heart leapt! The only way I could describe it is when you meet someone of the opposite sex and catching their eye your heart does a somersault! And each time you meet after that the same thing happens – well, I saw a photo, in this paper, and I fell in love with the photo of a bungalow in another part of Ashford. I wanted to ring the house agent there and then to see it ASAP! But what about Peter? Sometime before, when Chris was at home for a break, she suggested it might be a good idea if we moved into a bungalow. Peter's immediate reply was no, he wanted to stay in this house, (that we had been in since we married) until his dotage. Chris looked at me and asked what dotage meant. I said that I presumed he meant until he got carried out in his box! Peter nodded!

So, there was me wanting to phone a house agent about viewing a bungalow the other side of Ashford, and Peter's 'dotage' came to the front of my mind. So, what do I do? Well, what I would normally do in difficult situations – pray. So, I did: "What do I do Lord?" The answer was simple: "Show Peter the picture and ask him if he'd like to go and see it with you." Well, I had months before been and looked at a couple of bungalows in Willesborough where we lived. When I suggested Peter came and looked with me, he refused outright... the dotage thing I suppose some weeks before he gave that answer to Christine. So, I prayed if this was from God He would open the door. Now that I had handed it over, I had peace. So, when Peter got back from the day centre and we sat down with a cuppa and chatted about both our days, I grabbed the local paper, pointed out the picture of this bungalow, and asked him if he would like to go and see it with me. He looked at it for a few moments, and quietly said yes, he would. Thank You, Lord, I silently prayed. Whilst Peter was having a bit of a nap, I rang the agent in Ashford and asked if we could view that bungalow tomorrow, because Peter didn't have a day centre then. Yes, it was being viewed tomorrow afternoon at 3pm by a young couple vetting it for their elderly mother who fancied it, and they were dubious about it being suitable for a widow on her own. So, we would be very welcome to come and have a look at the same time. We could go around, just the two of us, and see what we think whilst the agent is talking to the young couple. Then we could speak to him when they left.

So, I checked on the way to get to this bungalow and drew a little map! Off we drove and just before 3pm, came in at the top of the road and drove very slowly down so as not to miss this rear-built bungalow on the right-hand side. I recognised it immediately from the newspaper photo and pulled into a space a few yards down in what was quite a narrow road. We got out, I took Peter's arm, crossed the road and we stood for a moment at the top of the drive with a large, detached house on the left, and a tiny bungalow on the right. We both looked down to a whitewashed bungalow at least one hundred yards at the end of the narrow drive. I took Peter's arm and down we went. When we got to the place which I recognised was the spot from which the agent's photo had been taken, my heart leapt again. Sometimes agents' photos are touched up to a certain degree. But they didn't need to here – this place will sell itself, on this warm, sunny July day! I loved the spaciousness, the lawns, the trees, the summer house, the garden seat on a lawn, a patio with potted plants, and what looked like a new conservatory attached to the right side of the building.

No one was in sight, I knew the owners weren't around that week, but I could hear voices, and the conservatory door was open. So, still holding Peter's hand, I called out and we stepped just inside. A smart suited man came immediately through the inside door of the conservatory, greeted us by name and introduced himself as the house agent. He explained he was showing around the family of the elderly lady interested in the bungalow. I said to him about the office saying they were a little dubious about their elderly mum buying the property and he confirmed that, and he was chatting to them, so they had the big picture. He invited Peter and I to look around inside on our own, and he would catch up with us when finished with the other folk. I threw up a little thank you prayer, because that was ideal with Peter with the dementia. To have a salesman showing us around and giving us the spiel in every room, would have overloaded Peter, and he would easily get anxious and confused, and could be troublesome. So, we wandered through the house at his pace. My love for this property was growing – everything had been done, even a lovely, fitted kitchen, and a new spacious bathroom extension. And I was already working out how I would use, and even rearrange the living areas and bedrooms. Peter was quiet and agreeable, and seemed, very peaceful for him, in such an unfamiliar situation.

The agent appeared again, and we had a brief chat and I indicated we were very interested. So, he suggested we had a good look around the garden; he would lock up the house, and we could, on this lovely summer day, linger as long as we wished and sit on the patio or the garden seat and just relax and enjoy the property in its peaceful position. And that's what we did.

Peter chose the garden seat in the middle of one of the lawns, facing the afternoon sun as it went around. We were on that property about an hour and a half, chatting on and off, but mainly enjoying the peaceful atmosphere.

When I asked him if he liked it, he immediately answered in the affirmative. I eventually managed to get him to move – it would be rush hour soon and I needed a few things from Sainsbury's.

Walking back up the drive to the road, a 'hullo' rang across from the vegetable garden at the side of the drive. It was a neighbour, a young woman about Christine's age. She asked if we were interested in the bungalow. I said yes and we exchanged a few pleasantries. She said: "You seem a lovely couple; I hope you get it! My name is Sue, by the way!"

Of course, I immediately replied; "I'm Sue too!"

"Oh great, hope to see you again then!"

I felt all the boxes were being ticked for us. So off we drove to Sainsbury's, and I knew my next move!

When we got to Sainsbury's I knew what to do. I asked Peter to go and get a trolley. Off he strolled, and I immediately rang the house agent, said who I was, and was asked how I got on at the bungalow. I answered in the affirmative and said: "I want to pay the full amount. Could you put things into motion please." Delighted, he said he would organise paperwork and contact me tomorrow for fuller details.

Next morning first thing I rang our bank adviser. Peter had been employed by the bank and had appointed us an adviser when they knew about the dementia. He had worked with us on several issues always in the beginning keeping Peter in the loop until he went into permanent care; then carrying on with Chris and myself, to work to a place where Peter's finances were sorted, for immediate need, long term care costs, and making sure I had enough income too.

It was more complicated than that, but I understood we were in safe hands and any fees were much smaller because Peter was a bank pensioner – one of the family. In this difficult and sometimes exhausting times, I had peace of mind for things were is safe hands.

The bank adviser rang the next morning to discuss the logistics of the move. I told him that I didn't want to sell one house and buy another. Firstly, I couldn't cope with buying and selling, as I was already exhausted caring for Peter, and I asked his advice. And Christine was considering returning home too.

We had a long discussion about it and he came up with a solution – using a trust fund left by an aunt of Peter's. It would act like a mortgage over the property, without usual payments, of course, and it would be restored to the trust fund if I sold the property, or if I died whilst still in the property.

CHAPTER 15

2013 – A BUSY YEAR OF CHANGE

WHAT A YEAR! So much change for the whole family as a whole and individually.

At the beginning it was the repeated attacks of bronchitis Peter suffered and Dr Joe telling me to take him somewhere warm for a month, and the wonderful four weeks in Gran Canaria with the children joining us for different weeks. What a blessed time that was for all of us, and the bronchitis stopped too!

But in April, Peter developed an inflamed lump on his leg. Dr Joe saw it, rang the hospital and we were up in a clinic within the hour. A thorough investigation confirmed Peter had a DVT in his leg, and six months of injections in his stomach started in that clinic. I was asked if I would take on the job of giving Peter the injection every day for six months starting there and then with the first one. I agreed and was very carefully instructed how to do it. Me doing the first one under instruction was much better for me than watching the nurse do the first one. I was much less nervous at home having done it that way.

May arrived and Ian, who lived in Harpenden, decided to apply to Ashford Borough Council for a single-person flat – he wanted to be nearer to be supportive as his dad's dementia developed. He was warned it could take eighteen months. Christine, living and working in Carlisle, was considering moving back to Ashford for the same reason and was coming down in May for a bit of a break with us. A friend in Carlisle told her she'd seen a job advertised in Ashford, Kent, that was just ideal for her – it had Chris' name on it! Chris investigated and liked what she saw and sent in her CV with her application form. They promptly replied to Chris to check if she was available immediately as they were arranging interviews. Oh dear, the first obstacle! She wasn't available until later in the summer when her present boss in Carlisle retired; there was a very busy workload in the following month and, as his PA, she just couldn't leave him in the lurch. They were sorry to have to leave her off the interview list. When Chris was with us the following week, she told us which day the interviews were being held for the Ashford job. Peter wasn't at this stage taking much in, but I had met the friend in Carlisle who thought the job was made for Chris, so I just quietly prayed: 'Lord, if that job is meant for Chris, keep the door open for her please!'

At 5.30pm Chris came in from her room with an email. It was from the interviewing team to say they had not appointed anyone suitable for the position. Chris was still the best qualified person for the job and they were willing to work around her schedule in Carlisle and get someone to cover until she was available if she could get down to Ashford as soon as possible and was successful in the interview. Wow, that was exciting! She emailed them to say she was in Ashford now with her parents, not very far from their office.

First thing next morning, they contacted her; could Chris come this lunchtime for an informal interview?

Yes!

She was away about four hours and came back with a smile on her face. It had been an intensive interview, and they were delighted to offer her the job and would work out together with her the best timing of it all. I smiled and sent up a silent prayer. From the moment that the Carlisle friend had seen the advert and told Chris it had her name on it... it was settled above before it was settled down here!

That was summer 2013, and she is still in that position now in 2021, albeit working from home for nearly a year because of the Covid pandemic, and her dad died in a local dementia care home in 2018 and went Home to Glory. That was the end of the long goodbye for Peter, and I am so grateful that he hadn't continued in that home into 2020, because I would be in the awful position of not being able to visit him now for nearly a year. My heart goes out to those with elderly relatives in homes and I have often shed tears at the thought of what they are going through.

Next to sort out in this busy year was the family holiday for four in Croatia booked a year before for the last week of September and the first week of October. Four now became two! Peter was out with the DVT, and Chris would have started her new job. That left Ian and me. Who shall we take with us! Well for me my local friend Lesley came immediately to mind. I always call her sister Joy, because that's the effect she always has on me! When I asked her, she was delighted to come. So, I had a chat with Ian, and he suggested his friend Aaron. I knew Aaron quite well, and he was a good friend to Ian. Aaron was delighted with the idea of a holiday together in Croatia. So, then I contacted Saga, who accepted the changes and would send out new paperwork. And indeed, it proved to be a great holiday for us all.

One dark cloud in this year of so many changes was with Archie, our lovely Springer Spaniel. He had developed a limp with a front leg but basic tests, x-rays and medicine for arthritis were not conclusive, and the latter made no difference to the limp. Also, he didn't seem to be in pain; but the limp became more pronounced. So, our vet got us up to a specialist in Bedfordshire. A friend drove us there and collected us the next day. Two days of consultations, in depth tests, some under anaesthetic meant Pete and I in a B&B. Thankfully we always have pet insurance!

The final consultation was not good news. It was much worse than arthritis. He turned the screen round to show us and told us Archie had a nerve plexus tumour. I asked what the white threads, like cotton, were. That was the

NPT tracking from its source in his front 'armpit'. I could see branches of it going in all directions. I pointed to one and he said that was tracking along the main nerve towards his trachea, his windpipe. There was no cure and he had left Archie under the anaesthetic, so we had the choice to leave him behind and let him go or take him home. Peter got very upset at this and shouted, "No, no!" That made the decision easier for me. I asked how long Archie would have. "Difficult to say – certainly weeks, maybe even two or three months at the most. You've had dogs before, haven't you Mrs Ross?" I nodded.

"Then you, and your vet will know the time to say goodbye." So, I looked to Pete and suggested the best thing was to take Archie home with us. He was calmer and agreed.

So, I thanked the consultant – he certainly was the expert in his field which we needed. BUT for the long goodbye of dementia that Peter, and I with him, were travelling, I would have made a clean break and left Archie under the anaesthetic which would have been increased until he gently stopped breathing. But more and more my priority was quality of life for Peter, with lots of love and care until his time came.

Next was our Croatia holiday and our friend, with two dogs, who usually has Archie for holidays said yes of course she would have him and give him the best of times even with this problem. And on our return, apart from the limp he was full of beans, as the saying goes;

and I had had a well needed break in Croatia, Peter had another respite time in the care home that sooner or later would be his permanent home; and Chris was settling well into her new job in Ashford.

We were now well into October of this year of change. It is amazing how a dog can teach you to live life to the full. And one incident comes to mind. It was, as far, as I recall, the last or one of the last times that Peter and I took Archie over Hothfield Common, and we were covering just the easier half of woods and fields. He was now on some arthritic medicine to keep any growing discomfort at bay, until....

We were in the top field walking towards the latched gate into the next field. Archie doing his usual spaniel, nose to the ground mode, didn't see the rabbit freeze this side of the gate at the sight of him. Peter and I saw it run to the left and stay very still amongst some thick ferns. Archie kept going to the gate, as we always did. Then, he caught a whiff of rabbit, stopped, looked to the left and saw it. No thought for his now partly paralyzed front leg, he moved, then the rabbit took off in circles to shake him off and finally through the undergrowth to the right of said gate. Phew! Well, the dog won't be able to follow him through that small space. So, Peter and I went through the gate too, but there was no sight or sound of our Archie. So, we called and called and looked around the area keeping the gate in view. I was beginning to have a sinking feeling that maybe he had chased the bunny through the wood and even as far as the busy road. Oh no, the thought was broken by a rustling and

Archie appeared with the rabbit, intact, in his mouth. He dropped down exhausted beside a tree and didn't move as I walked slowly toward him.

"What a clever dog you are!" No way was I going to tell him off; in his condition he did an amazing thing! I felt proud of him – hope that doesn't offend anyone reading this!

"Are you going to let me see your prize, Archie? Show me." I put my hand out. He immediately put his treasure down in front of me, and simply allowed me to pick it up. There were no wounds on it – it probably died of fright when caught.

"It's yours Archie, you keep it."

Peter never said a word, just watched and listened. I took his hand and said: "We will walk slowly. Archie knows the route well enough by now!"

So, we walked and over the next twenty minutes, around the top of the field, down through another gate, down the slope to the stream, and up the first part of the steep path through the wood that would get us eventually back to the car park – three times Archie overtook us, to flop down ahead of us with less and less rabbit to be eaten, more and more in the bulging stomach of our dog. Finally, he appeared, wobbling like a fat lady, with the whole rabbit inside, and taking the slope very slowly.

A thought struck me as I witnessed this sight, and I voiced what I was thinking: "Archie, you are not getting in my car and throwing all that up as we drive home!"

So, we zigzagged back and forth, in and out the wood and field. But obviously Peter had had enough excitement and we went back to the car park with a silent prayer that Archie would wait till he got home before he thew that rabbit up! Amazingly that rabbit was never seen again. I put dog, with rabbit, in the garden for at least an hour and he slept it off!

We didn't actually move into the bungalow until the end of November, but the 'adventures' of a busy 2013 continued at times to take us by surprise – there never seemed to be an uneventful day! Was that when my greying hair turned white!!

Towards the end of October I was browsing on the internet and came across a site called 'Preloved'. I can't say any sections interested me until I found myself flicking over pictures of dogs, which would always interest me! So, I stopped and there in front of me was a picture of two Springers. I showed Chris and she remarked how good it has been having a dog around for dad with the dementia. What! I knew Archie's days were very much numbered, but to have two new lively Springers, with our old dog dying, and dad with dementia – that seemed an awful lot to cope with. But with Chris back in Ashford and settling into her new job I had support now in situ. I kept looking at the photos of these two dogs, Bonnie and Clyde, owned by a man in

Maidstone whose situation had changed drastically, and who needed genuine experienced dog lovers to adopt them and give them the home they deserved. They were brother and sister, properly trained and very happy, well-behaved dogs needing a loving home. In the end I knew I would regret it in the not-too-distant future if I didn't at least contact their owner, Steve.

Hearing we were just up the road in Ashford, He arranged to drive over the next afternoon. Of course, I was not surprised to open the door and see those spaniel eyes looking at me. We had had Springers since 1985 and the eyes have it, and I have rescued them ever since. Steve had brought his little girl with the dogs. I saw those two dogs get out of their car and come up my drive without leads on. He had trained them well. We had a chat, and the dogs had a look around. My most vivid memory I still can see was our Archie curled up in his bed in front of the fireplace. He looked up at the visitors but stayed in his bed.

THEN, Bonnie, the bitch who had had two litters of babies apparently – she stopped next to Archie still curled up in his bed, sniffed him thoroughly, and then slowly and gently she eased herself into this one dog bed and carefully wrapped herself around Archie, who didn't move. It IS a well-known fact that some dogs can sniff out cancer, and obviously Springers are used as sniffer dogs in many different scenarios. It fairly brought tears to my eyes to see Bonnie do that; I think that was the iconic moment for me to make the decision to adopt these two dogs.

Next the little girl, Ruby, got a packet of dog treats and sat up on our settee, and called the dogs saying "treats!" I am not kidding – her two dogs were there in a trice, and she was having no nonsense – they had to sit, wait, and be still. A few seconds later Archie had climbed out of bed and squeezed himself between the visiting dogs. And I have a photo somewhere of these three pooches, rigidly to attention, no shoving and pushing! She fed them a little treat out of the bag, one at a time, slowly. When she said they were all gone, they lay down, and Archie went back into his bed.

We all agreed – Steve wanted us to adopt his two gorgeous spaniels, and we said yes, we'd love to. He arranged to come back next day with them, and all the stuff we would need, leads, collars, balls and toys, bowls and all the paperwork, especially vet records and kennel Cub stuff.

Next afternoon I had a plan. When Steve arrived with the two additions to our family and all their bibs and bobs, I asked Steve if he would like to come over to see the property we were soon to move into, where his Bonnie and Clyde would be living soon. Yes, he jumped at that. So, I rang the bungalow and the present owner answered; she was sitting on the patio in the sun, and yes of course we could come over with the dogs. So, Steve followed us in his car with the dogs. He followed us down the narrow drive to the bungalow, parked the car and got out, saying: "Is this all your garden?" I nodded, then waved to the house owner, and she told us to help ourselves. So, Steve let the dogs out of the boot and they

78

were off excitedly exploring everywhere! They loved it, and so did Steve! All their stuff was in the car. I said: "Get their ball out of the car Steve, I want to show you something." So, he did and tossed it up the garden and they chased after it and dropped it at his feet. So, I told him to hold onto it and follow me. I led them down to the back gate and it wasn't until I opened it that he realised.

"Your back gate leads onto a field! Wow, I thought the garden was big... and this as well!" The dogs were bouncing around obviously wanting him to throw their ball out here!

"Watch this," Steve said. He called the dogs to heel with them sitting, in front of him, and facing the opposite side of the field. He made them 'stay' for what seemed a lifetime. Then he threw it high and across the field nearly to the other side. Those two dogs never moved, except their heads lifted as they watched the ball all the way until it landed right over to the far side. Still, they never moved. I was beginning to get a real good idea of how well he had trained these dogs. Then he shouted "fetch!" and they were off like greyhounds. Alpha dog Clyde got there by a whisker, and they both came back wagging their tails. This was to be their forever home, for I had fallen in love with those gorgeous dogs – and I got a bonus too! We had a quick chat with the soon-to-move owner of the bungalow, and thanked her, and we drove back home, Steve and the dogs behind us. He unloaded his car of doggy stuff, said his goodbyes to them and left, happy that they were going to a home they would love, and he asked if he could visit in the future once we were settled in the bungalow. Of course.

Archie was clearly an 'end-of-life' dog, more noticeable with the two youngsters around. But they were so good with him, and he seemed to find comfort in their company too and I was so glad I overlapped. But he was sleeping a lot more and was on medication. The vet said if there was any noticeable change, I should bring him in. Peter was on a short respite break when one day Chris and I looked at each other and we knew. We rang the vet, and he gave us a time to bring him in by the back door. I always hold my dogs when we come to this time. I know folk who cannot cope with seeing their pet put to sleep leave it all to the vet, and I would never criticise such a personal decision. This time I wasn't alone. We stayed with Archie holding him and talking to him until he was gone. Then we were led out the back door and down the steps both crying. Chris was first to speak: "We've got two dogs at home, let's collect them and take them for a long walk over Hothfield Common." That's what we did, and what a difference it made. I had always left gaps between dogs; this was the first time I overlapped. And I so appreciated these two super Springers who took the edge off the grief of losing Archie.

We finally moved into the bungalow on 30th November, 2013. We put the dogs in kennels for two days and the day after a neighbour came down to help move all the boxes into the spare bedroom so we could move normally around the property and deal with a box at a time. That helped Peter settle initially, and I was so relieved that there were no stairs for him to tumble down ever again – a great weight off my mind. Having said that, the dementia moves on, progressing along an unpredictable course. He had started to wander out in the street in the old house, usually looking for me. I might be collecting a prescription, or in the corner shop, but he would wander out even in the rain and in his slippers. But usually if I told him where I was going and left him a note to read, he was fine for a while. I would take him with me where I could, and Ian, now living in a flat in Ashford, would cycle over and stay with his dad sometimes when I went out, and always leave Peter phone numbers to ring. All these things worked for a while until the next stage of the long goodbye of this awful disease.

But we managed Christmas in the bungalow – it was quiet with Chris away on a sabbatical break until the New Year. So, Ian came to stay and he liked to have all the fun of a traditional Christmas, and his dad enjoyed all the distractions too – decorations, presents, festive food, and two lovely spaniels!

I did wonder if 2013 would be Peter's last Christmas living at home… but changes came quicker than I anticipated.

CHAPTER 16

DEMENTIA GRIP TIGHTENS

DURING DECEMBER 2013 and into January 2014 the progress of the dementia in Peter's brain was showing more and more signs of intruding into different areas of his life and affecting the functions in parts of his body. At the top of the list was unpredictability. By now I couldn't go out, leave him in alone, not even when I went out to collect a prescription five minutes away. The last occasion that I did, I got back, got out of the car, and I could hear a man's voice in the kitchen talking to Peter, and the telly in the living room had been switched on. I went in and there was Jim, a near neighbour, chatting to Peter and making them both a cup of tea. He explained to me that he had been in his front garden and coming onto the pavement to tidy up his hedge when he saw Peter appear at the top of our long drive, turn left and walk up towards the main road. He called his name and caught up with him and asked him if he was all right and where was he going. The answer was that he was trying to catch up with Sue! Jim did understand from Peter that I had said not to leave the house and I would be back soon. So, being December, albeit a sunny day, and Peter in slippers and no coat, Jim suggested they went back to the bungalow together and have nice hot cup of tea and wait for Sue! One thing Peter loved was a nice cup of tea! So, they both went back together, and that's where I found them – the telly on and Peter just settled down watching it with his cuppa when I turned up. Jim and I had a short chat. I thanked him very much, said I knew we were getting to a point with the dementia when I would not be able to leave him alone again at all. It's been coming gradually, and this was it.

I was and still am a sound sleeper. Once I am asleep not even a thunderstorm disturbs me! My lightest sleep is, I suppose, the hour before I become fully awake. One night, well actually the morning before 7am, I was gradually pulled into consciousness by Peter's voice shouting: "Help me, help me someone!"

Again: "Help me, I am trapped, someone help me." I guessed that he couldn't now always remember me, to call me. But as soon as I was fully awake, I jumped out of bed, went to my door and opened it. He was between the easy chair and the wall in the living room. It was the chair I usually sat in to watch telly in the evening. Peter sat in a similar chair to the left of mine with a little table in between. So, I spoke his name and he looked at me blankly which would be an increasing sign of the dementia. It wasn't yet properly light and of course the curtains were still drawn, although I had a set of mini portable lights that ran on three Duracell batteries. You could put them on flat surfaces to give light in a room without disturbing sleep; or pull off the paper on the back and stick them on doors, for example to give light directions to the toilet – which is what I did. But Peter had come out of his room and felt he was stuck. So, I took his hand and led him out through the gap I often used to go between my chair and the radiator to get to my room. I put the main light on and showed him where he had been 'trapped'. He thanked me for rescuing him! Another characteristic of the long goodbye of dementia is the regression back to childhood ways. And I saw a lot of that when I became a regular visitor at the dementia care home.

That last incident was basically confusion, one or the earlier characteristics of someone developing this disease. Another one, the same week I slept through, I didn't hear a thing. When I got up, dressed, and went to the bathroom, the door on the left, (before the bathroom straight ahead with a light and label), was open and everything in that utility room was trashed, looking like a bomb had hit it. I used the bathroom and went back to Peter's room. He was still asleep and snoring! He must have had an active night! So, I went back to the kitchen and started laying the table for breakfast. Peter came in looking tired.

"You look tired Pete; have you been dreaming?"

"No," he said, "someone imprisoned me and wouldn't let me out. I did shout but you didn't hear me. I got out eventually."

I took him next door to the utility room, and he looked. Yes, that was it. So, I gently explained that there was no intruder in the house the previous night, that he mistook the door to the utility room for the bathroom, and pointed to the bathroom with the label and the little light on it, still on. He was okay with all that and came into the kitchen to have some breakfast with me.

Those two incidents, which were 'confusion', weren't repeated. But other night-time incidents, in those first two weeks of the NEW year 2014, were more serious. I didn't know then but discovered later that year that they were known under the heading ASC – Altered State of Consciousness, which was in the list of testing criteria for NHS Continuing Care assessments.

The first incident was again in the middle of the night. I didn't hear Peter come into my room, but him crashing against the filing cabinet next to the door did wake me and I saw him with a torch in his hand. I called out: "Are you okay Pete, the light is by the door." He put the light on but didn't say a word. He walked across towards the window where there was a green bin, for rubbish, with a lid on it, and lined with a black bin liner – fortunately, for he took the lid off, dropped it on the floor and proceeded to wee in the bin.

"No Pete, that's not a toilet, that's my bin for rubbish."

"No, it IS the toilet," was his short reply and he left and went back to his room and closed the door.

I got up, took the bin to the bathroom, got rid of the wee, and tied up the black sac and put it in the bath and into the black refuse bin next morning. I then put another liner and screwed up newspaper in the bin and next day I took it into Peter's room, beside his bed, and told him he could wee in there if he needed to during the night. The phrase comes to mind eight years later, as I write this: 'If you can't beat them, join them!' But at the time I was on a learning curve to be with Peter where he was at all the stages that we had ahead of us together, of this long goodbye. And yes, he did use it as a wee pot in his bedroom.

The second example of this Altered State of Consciousness was within days of the last one. Again, it was at night, and this time it certainly woke me up. A torch was shining in my face, a deep threatening voice growling at me: "What are you doing in my bed? Get out, get out!" And the bed clothes were whipped off me. I flicked my bedside light on and looked into the face of my husband. He wasn't sleepwalking; his eyes were staring angrily at me and in a second, I knew instinctively not to question or disagree. As I swung my legs out of the bed on the other side, I threw up a quick prayer and felt at peace immediately.

"I am sorry Pete, could you help me back to MY room," and I walked towards the door ahead of him, and he followed. Once in the living room I saw he had left his light on in his room. "Oh, there's a light in the room over there, let's go and see." The room we had just left was the coldest room in the bungalow. It was the most recent extension, and had three outside walls, and was a great size for an office/bedroom. I loved it. As we stepped into Peter's bedroom, I felt the warmth and exclaimed to him behind me: "Actually Pete, this room is so much warmer than yours back there." I quickly moved to the bed and felt the still warm bedclothes. "Peter, feel this bed, it's lovely and warm too. Would you feel more comfortable here in the warm, and swap with me?" He put his hand on the bed beside my hand, and simply replied: "Yes." I said: "Your hand feels cold Pete; keep your dressing gown on and let me help you into bed and tuck you in." Without a murmur he got into bed, I straightened his dressing gown and the duvet, and kissed him goodnight, leaving just the little side light on and turning off the main light.

I went back to my own bedroom, had a short time of prayer thanking God for giving me His Peace and His Wisdom.

I slept soundly and when I woke up, I quietly looked in on Peter who was soundly asleep as I had left him.

CHAPTER 17

THE FUTURE IS MAPPED OUT

I DIDN'T NORMALLY WRITE a diary but more and more I was jotting in a notebook or on pieces of paper, not very organised I must admit. But I began to feel that one day I would write a second book and it would be on this most feared disease with no cure – DEMENTIA. For already at this stage, I was on a steep learning curve about something I had no previous experience of at all. So, every stage with Peter was another stage of knowledge and understanding, and at times absolute revelation to me. AND of course, each stage brought its challenges, especially as the person I was walking the walk with was my own dear husband.

A couple of days after that last disturbed night with Peter having an episode of ASC, I sat staring at my computer. I couldn't focus on anything. I felt so exhausted. I did the safest thing I know – I turned to God in prayer. 'Lord, I feel exhausted; I have chosen to care for Peter for as long as possible despite the advice of doctors and nurses, particularly at the hospital. I have always known that a time would come when the only choice is for him to go into a dementia care or nursing home. You have given me such peace during some scary incidents with him. But he is at such an advanced stage now Lord, and I am so exhausted; I can't go on much longer. BUT, but Lord, and it's a big BUT – I can't make the decision to put him into Warren Lodge, who have cared for him on respite breaks and will welcome him back fulltime when the time comes. Lord, I just can't make the decision. To do that I feel that I will be abandoning him. I simply can't do it. So, I am handing it all over to You Lord, and asking that You take over.'

I cried as I prayed this…. and I am crying as I write it. But I did the best that I could, I let go, and carried on caring for my husband,

The next day Christine rang just to say she was safely back from her two-month sabbatical in Australia and New Zealand. We were looking forward to speaking soon and updating on all the news.

Not long after that brief call Peter came to me. I was about to say Chris is home safe, but he started talking to me, but I couldn't understand what he was saying. So, I asked him to repeat it slowly what he was trying to say. And he did speak slowly, and he thought he was telling me something, but there was no way it was English or any language for that matter. But he seemed in real earnest to let me know something. So, I took that seriously with a quick arrow prayer.

Immediately an idea – I picked up a pen and notepad and asked him to write down what he was saying. I stayed where I was and gave him room to write at the end of the table. From where I was, I could see he was writing a couple of sentences. When he handed back what he had written I was shocked. Yes, it looked like a sentence of words of different lengths but was to me a jumble of letters that he thought were words. The two things – he couldn't speak properly, or write anything legible, and one thing immediately came to mind – a mini stroke or TIA for short. I said: "Let's have a cuppa, Pete; I'll put the kettle on and go to the loo. Come and sit down in your easy chair." I took the piece of paper and my phone with me, switched the kettle on and went into the bathroom, closed the door and rang Chris back, told her what I thought it was and she said to ring for an ambulance. I did that and they came promptly, checked Peter over and said they would take him to the hospital. Did I want to come in the ambulance or would I follow in the car? I said that I would follow to A&E in the car.

In A&E a TIA was confirmed; a consultant from the stroke clinic assessed him as safe to go home and gave me an appointment for him at stroke outpatients in three days' time, January 15th, 2014.

We arrived on time at stroke outpatients. We had about fifteen minutes' wait, and Peter was quite fidgety, which was becoming the status quo when we had appointments. In some ways dementia sufferers revert or regress to behaviour more and more like little children again. And once we had been shown in to see the consultant, Peter wouldn't stop fidgeting! So, the man in charge called a tall, well-built Sister in: "Sister, would you take Mr Ross for a nice walk down the corridor please?" Peter willingly went with Sister! And in all his years in dementia care he was always walking somewhere, outside, inside, down the corridors, into the garden. They even found him in the car park once – how? Well, that's another story.

So back to my chat with the consultant. He got straight to the point: "Mrs Ross, or can I call you Suzanne?" I nodded. "I would like to keep Peter in for a few days for medical and psychiatric assessment with a view to him going straight into dementia residential nursing care. The dementia is far too advanced for him to be cared for at home any longer. Do I have your agreement on this?" I felt my defences rise on Peter's behalf, and was about to object, when I felt what was like a gentle tap on the shoulder and a voice that only I heard said: "Sue, you asked Me to take over."

It was as though a ton weight fell off my shoulders in that moment. I nodded: "Yes I agree, thank you." So, Peter was given a bed in the Clinical Decision ward for a series of tests and assessments. A couple of days later I saw Dr Andrew, the psychiatrist who had eventually diagnosed Peter with dementia several years back now! She was lovely; she took quite a long time with me giving me updated information, explaining what tests they were doing and answering all of my questions. She did say she believed Peter had had multiple TIAs, and the dementia was now very advanced. The next day the hospital social services dept wanted to do an assessment known as a Continuing Care Assessment to see if Peter now qualified for the NHS to pay his fees in the dementia care home. The psychiatrist and the Social Services manager both felt confident that he would qualify. But all the results for CC assessment went to a full CC committee meeting.

On January 20th, 2014, Peter was transferred directly to Warren Lodge Dementia Care Nursing home. The CC Committee fast tracked their answer – no, Peter did not qualify at this time.

The hospital Social Services Manager, who had seen the results of a previous assessment when Peter was in hospital after his fall downstairs and the broken pelvis, and this new assessment, could see that the latest one showed how much of a deterioration had happened in Peter's condition.

She was furious and said that I must appeal the result, and as Peter's Power of Attorney I had the authority to do that. Our son, Ian, who had seen a fair amount of his dad over these months also told me to appeal.

But after holding myself together looking after Peter to this point, when he was safely in the care of Warren Lodge, the accumulated exhaustion hit me like a ton of bricks.

He was now safe; and I knew I must give myself time to fully recover before I engaged in what I had begun to realise would be a battle of a different kind. I needed a break. I knew the senior nurse on duty in Warren Lodge. He had previously been involved in the hospital, with the psychiatrist on a course for dementia sufferers and their spouses. I was in Warren Lodge to see Peter settled on his first day. And this wise nurse, Norman, told me he needed time to settle in, and I needed time to recover my mojo. How long did he recommend? Two weeks. I accepted that and, in a sense, had a two-week vacation just five minutes' drive from Peter's new home.

CHAPTER 18

DEMENTIA IS A HEALTHCARE NEED, NOT SOCIAL

WITH PETER now in safe care, even though it took some months to get over the exhaustion, I was now having quality time visiting, without the responsibility of being his full-time carer. I also enjoyed getting to know the staff and realised it was a comprehensive group of people that made up a whole team... manager, reception and office, nurses and their team of carers, activities team, the chef who brought scrummy food down, and the hidden hard workers in the kitchen and the laundry room. It wasn't perfect because no one is perfect, but the more time I was in there the more I appreciated what was done for Peter and two floors of primarily dementia sufferers.

By the end of May 2014, I had fully recovered from the exhaustion and was ready to get down to business. I wrote a series of letters. The first, early June, was to the senior person at the top of the Kent NHS Continuing and funded Nursing Care. I was now appealing, as advised in January, against the decision to refuse Peter Continuing Care when tested before his direct transfer from William Harvey Hospital to Warren Lodge, top floor.

I was now acutely aware that Peter's monthly fee for the privilege of being in dementia care at that time was £5000 per month.

I also wrote letters to the Prime Minister at 10 Downing Street, the health minister at the Health Dept, the newly appointed head of the NHS, who had, to kick off his term in office, written an article in a national daily paper that I read every day, that his top priority was to sort out the unfair and uneven system relating to dementia sufferers having to pay private nursing home rates. I was so encouraged by that. And finally, I wrote to my Ashford MP, Damian Green. Apart from him I am not naming names because they are all history now as I write this in 2021, except for Damian who is still in office as Ashford's MP.

The Prime Minister replied – he thanked me for bringing the whole matter to his attention and had passed the details of my letter onto the health minister. The latter replied in detail about the status quo concerning the 'care' system, especially the inequalities in the support and care of the elderly, including dementia. He acknowledged that although some small changes can be made more promptly, there was a real need to overhaul the whole system which would take a lot more time and cooperation over the whole of parliament, and with the NHS and local councils. And he thanked me for the very valid points I had made concerning dementia sufferers paying high private fees even though it is a terminal condition with no cure.

What about the new head of the NHS? The page he filled in a national newspaper gave me great hope, but to no avail. He was the only one out of the four top servants of the people of this land, who never replied at all. What a disappointment, to put it lightly.

The last one on the list I wrote to was the best of the lot. Damian Green, our local MP, contacted me several times. He thanked me for my letter and would indeed investigate it. He asked for more specific details about Peter's situation; he sympathised with me and understood where I was coming from, because his own father had dementia. He asked me if I could come and see him at his surgery – he lived in a village outside Ashford. Christine wanted to go with me, and he made us both very welcome. Very relaxed time on two visits, and he made us feel that our personal situation with Peter mattered to him. He was and is a good local MP. We were impressed. He spent a lot of time for us, and with us. But in the end the local situation on dementia care was no worse or better than elsewhere in the country as far as the present system went, and what was needed most was a total change in the whole care system in our land.

This would be a huge change and as always it comes down to finances. Meanwhile he encouraged us to push on with obtaining Continuing Care for Peter, and not give up. And his door was always open; if we wanted to see him again just ring his secretary for an appointment.

Things settled down for Peter in Warren Lodge into his first summer there, and I got into a routine visiting during the week several afternoons and together with the children over the weekends. I had no immediate answer to my letter to the leader of the Continuing Care. Norman the senior nurse rang CC, also sometime in May to tell them that Peter had deteriorated in several areas and now needed continuing care. I was there when he rang. They said they would get back to Warren Lodge and arrange a meeting and fresh assessment. On July 8th they hadn't replied to my May letter or to the senior nurse's request.

New management came into place that week, the deputy covering had had no response, and on the 15th the new manager said to leave it in her hands. Peter had had falls and was refusing medication, and she was going to pursue continuing care assessment for him. Eventually a continuing care assessment was scheduled in late August. Peter had had several falls early to mid-August and was in A&E twice. The most recent of those falls happened in the dining room in front of the manager, and the activities leader who told me that as she was speaking to Peter, his eyes went fixed and blank, and he went down forwards like a pole... unconscious. Fortunately chairs and tables broke his fall, and moments later they helped him back onto his feet. There was agreement that he likely had a TIA, which we knew had happened before several times.

A couple of days later the long-awaited continuing care assessment day arrived, and both Chris and I decided to attend together.

I sensed immediately that we were not in the presence of a sympathetic person. The leaders of these meetings are usually qualified nurses who have been trained, well trained, in this specific work of continuing care assessment, and previous ones we met with, were professional, calm, sympathetic of the emotional situations we, as next of kin, were in, and the previous one had a lovely, gentle, compassionate way of dealing with us too.

But this woman assessor was different. From the start she seemed to want to get on with the business and I felt we were being dragged along. There was a Warren Lodge staff member with us for some of the time, but who got called away. I am usually quite relaxed in most situations, but the way she was rollercoasting her way through this assessment, that we had waited many months for, was stressing me and I was getting a headache. Chris too had said little at that stage.

I decided on a very recent incident – the one where Peter went down like a ton of bricks, where, in the dining room he was included in the conversation between the Home Manager and the Activities Manager. They got him up and sat him down, and that should have been put in his notes immediately. I shared this with the increasingly unsympathetic woman. Her immediate reply was that it had not been recorded; when I said one of those managers had shared it with me. She said that what I reported didn't count, only what was recorded in the home's notes and records. At that Christine strongly objected; of course, her mother's relevant reports counted.

The response was again in the negative. Chris looked close to tears; me too, and my head was thumping. We just let the session come to the brief end that this assessor had been aiming for from the beginning.

We left feeling like we had been pulled through a hedge backwards. The manager wasn't in her office when we left, but I knew I had to speak to her. Chris and I went to our cars and on the opposite side of the carpark was the assessor chatting and laughing with a woman I didn't recognise. The tears came again as we parted – Chris back to work, and me back home. Neither of us wanted to go through another of those assessments again.

I saw the manager the next day and shared with her and she was quite upset about it. She said that discussions had been going on, and there was going to be a change with the way assessments were done in the home.

I was always informed but never went to another assessment until what turned out to be the last one as Peter had been put into 'end of life' care and given three days. The assessor was so lovely; she had gone to see Peter in bed, then came back and started an assessment in the familiar order, with the home nurse present. She didn't get far, decided to abort the assessment; the nurse agreed, and she immediately awarded Peter a successful Continuing Care Assessment, opened her computer and signed it off there and then with the virtual signatures of the nurse and myself alongside hers.

I asked her when that was effective from and how much would Peter be left paying. She said it was effective from NOW, AND the full amount that Peter had been paying would now be paid by the government (NHS and Social Services). I gave her a hug!

I received a phone call the next morning before my breakfast, from an official confirming that Peter would no longer be paying anything for his care. I appreciated his call very much. It sealed the reality for me.

 In January 2014 Peter started paying £5000 monthly for his care, and his last payment in July 2017 was £5,700 monthly. There is still no cure for dementia – it is a terminal disease and a very cruel one; and today, in 2021, Boris Johnson's government has just once again kicked this political football back into touch.

CHAPTER 19

IN-HOUSE LESSONS ALONG THE JOURNEY

IN THE EARLY DAYS of Peter's final years in the dementia home there was much that was unfamiliar to cause him more confusion, and for me so much to learn that was all very new to me.

At first, when I visited him, he was pleased to see me, and I him. The downside was when I was ready to leave, he was up like a shot and running after me from the lounge to the lift. It wasn't unusual in those early days to have up to five staff members holding on to him so I could get in the lift to go to the ground floor. I knew it wouldn't be helpful to any of us if I gave in and went back in with him for a little longer.

A few visits on, we were relaxing in the lounge together with a cuppa and cake. By this time I was well aware of the cost of his stay which was eye watering, and I was well aware by now that the only way this would be free would be if and when he was awarded Continuing Care. I realised that in those early days, despite caring for him myself until his dementia was advanced too far for me to care for him any longer, he had to be end-of-life before he was paid for by the state. So, I let this go, and was grateful for the care he did have, and I was fully restored from exhaustion and was able to enjoy my visits to him, and go home to the bungalow and take Bonnie and Clyde, my Springers, out for a run.

So over our cup of tea that afternoon I said to Pete: "Do you realise how much you are paying for your stay here, Pete?" He had worked in investment banking for 40 years and was a man who really knew how to handle money and make it grow! But his dementia had advanced too, and I was testing his responses to what was a huge part of his life's work. His answer to the above question was a slow relaxed: "Nooo!"

I continued: "Do you want to know how MUCH you are charged here?"

Again, a slow and relaxed: "Yees!"

Without hesitation I replied: "£5000 per month."

"Ooh," was again the relaxed reply from my husband, the ex-banker.

"You are not worried about it, are you, Pete?"

"Noo," was again his slow relaxed reply.

My heart did a flip; wow, my husband all those years I had known him, with all that banking training, had always been concerned and felt overly responsible about finances; and he had no reason to be – he was very successful in his job and very astute with the finances.

Why do I share this?

It was the first POSITIVE I saw in dementia; and to see positives in dementia, that cruel destroyer of the brain, with no cure, lifted my spirit.

I drove home talking to the Lord Jesus: 'Thank you Lord for that; to see a positive in dementia to me is a miracle. Please open my eyes along this journey now with Pete, to see more miracles along the way. Thank you, Lord.' Now I felt I was on an adventure and there was more to come, and I wasn't walking alone along this journey with Peter.

The next 'positive' came a few weeks later. I usually walked the dogs twice in the day before my visits to Peter in the afternoons, usually about four a week. But some days when I also had appointments, or my Sainsbury's big shop, and I also visited Peter, then I would feel quite tired. I would sit next to him in an easy chair, chat a little and just BE. He seemed very relaxed, so I put my hand over his hand and relaxed beside him. Within a couple of minutes, when I looked over, I realised he was asleep. I took the opportunity and closed my eyes too. After a minute or so I opened my eyes and I saw two carers working nearby grinning at Peter and me! When I asked them what was funny, they quietly said that I had been asleep about half an hour! I was amazed, and I felt refreshed. Peter didn't wake up at this but continued deeply asleep. The carer nearest nodded to the door. Would it work, I thought? I lifted my hand slowly off his, and he continued gently snoring. It worked – there was no sign of him running after me at the lift and fighting off five carers to get to me. A quick thank you prayer as I got into the car, wondering if that was a one-off.

No, it wasn't. In future visits, when I was ready to go, I would put my hand over his, whispered my love for him, and closed my eyes. I would feel him relax immediately at what was obviously a comforting touch and word from me. And always in just two or three minutes, he was asleep.

So, I continued to thank God for showing me positives in this very long goodbye that is dementia.

More Lord!

CHAPTER 20

MY FREEDOM GREW IN THE CARE HOME

THOSE FIRST TWO POSITIVES gave the beginning of a walk in that place, that was to be a walk of freedom, that changed the way I was, and felt about dementia, the home, the other residents, the staff and what I saw of people at different stages of the disease that would sooner or later take their lives.

Fear and dark thoughts disappeared. I was alive; I felt free, and I would, particularly if Peter had dosed off, move around and chat to members of staff, and residents. Certainly, I felt that staff needed encouragement and a bit of normal banter from outside the world they worked in; a lot of them were on twelve-hour shifts. But whilst the staff were busy in and out working hard, the residents were settled in easy chairs in the lounge area, and moved a few yards in the open plan area, into the dining area for meals.

No two residents were the same – they were all unique individuals, despite the levelling effect of the dementia on them. Even that was different too with each person. Being a teacher by training, my head enjoyed being in learning mode a lot of the time. Sometimes observing new residents settling in I was having a guess at what work they did in their pre-dementia years. The first little lady I observed was always very busy in the lounge-dining room area. She was always busy, using the flat of her hand wiping across tables, chairs, under people's saucers, and even the floor. I guessed she had been a cleaner in her working life. So, when I had the opportunity I would ask the nurse-in-charge what work that lady had done. Apparently, she had worked as a cleaner and a waitress for many years!

Then there was the tall thin often agitated lady. I would sit down and talk to her. She was quite a quick talker and seemed very busy. I asked her if I could help; she immediately said yes; she had arranged a meeting for 5.30pm that day and could I arrange for a taxi to pick up four people at the station at 5 o'clock to come here. Yes, I could do that.

I saw the nurse on the way out and pointed out to her the most recent resident. I told her the job she'd asked me to do, and asked her what work this lady had done, as she seemed to me to have been some sort of boss who was stressed at not being in control of things in this new place; obviously her dementia was not as advanced as many others. Apparently, she had been in management on land, and then as a lover of ocean cruises, had taken up the post on a large cruise ship, as overall team manager responsible for the whole range of activities on the ship – daytime and night-time activities. A big responsibility, and potentially stressful – any problems and the buck stopped at her door. And having chatted to her early on, I was now enlisted in her team! And as someone coming in from the outside, she often asked me to arrange taxis for folk coming to conferences with her! Fortunately, her memory over days was at dementia level, so when I visited Peter later in the week, she had forgotten she had asked me! Most visitors stayed with their own relatives, but I got to love the folk in there as I chatted often to whoever was seated either side of Peter. And as he did more dosing I would often go around and say hullo to other residents and some of their visitors. Peter had been there about two years when a nurse said to me: "Sue, you ought to get a job here… you would be good." I took it as a compliment, but my answer was immediate: "Not likely, with my husband in here!"

I had no idea then that over two and a half years later, two months after Peter died, I did just that! More of that later.

But I can't move on without mentioning Joan. I can use the name because there were so many Joans in there – I guess it was the most popular girl's name in the pre-war generation, now those in their eighties or even nineties! I soon realised that Joan never had visitors, but I got to understand why. Joan was usually sitting in the dining room area when I arrived, and I would go to the serving area to make myself a cuppa and snaffle one of the chef's delicious cakes!

If Peter was in the loo or had gone for a wander, I would stop near where Joan was sitting at a table. I would first say hullo to Joan and then watch her eyes; I had learned to be careful near her because if she fancied, she would hurl a cup at you! So, either I kept my distance, said hello and kept going; or I would sit opposite her at the table and chat for a short time. The part of Joan's brain that dementia had affected most was language. In fact, I only heard three things come out of her mouth, with such a loud voice that a town crier would have been proud of! The most common two phrases that bellowed out of her mouth were always shouted together. For propriety's sake I will use a few stars! When I came into the room and she saw me, I would always greet her: "Hello, Joan, how are you?"

A pregnant pause was followed by a loud: "You're a big s**t, you're a f***ing c***!" For a long time, that's all she said to me, and it was also all I heard coming from her room when carers were in there helping her. And the only other thing I heard her say in her one and only town crier volume, when she had dropped or thrown her cup on the floor: "Can I have another cup of tea please?"

So how did I react to this, considering that no one had ever used such colourful language at me before? Well from the outset it made me smile, and after a while I realised, I just felt love for her, and when I realised this, what I said to her, each time she shouted these **** at me, I said, accompanying my smile: "Joan, I love you!"

She looked at me silently as I got up to join Pete, whether he was in the lounge or occasionally in his room in the early days. As the years went by, I always responded to the**** language with: "I love you, Joan." It always quietened her. Somewhere deep inside her she knew I meant it. A postscript – she was still going strong when Peter died. At his funeral one of the home's managers came with a beautiful testimony to Peter from the senior nurse, who had been there all the time he was. I went over to thank her for bringing it, and she caught my arm and told me that Joan had asked several times: "Where is Sue?" Obviously, I asked which Joan because there were a number of them! She confirmed it was Joan with the **** language. I was in disbelief because to my knowledge Joan never knew or used my name. Her reply was that Joan did know my name and was missing me. As she shared that with me, we were both close to tears. I hugged her and thanked her – I was SO blessed that she shared that with me. But most all I thanked God that He gave me a real love for that Joan, who never had any visitors because family and old friends simply couldn't cope with the way the dementia had cruelly affected Joan.

PS. I believe that Joan once knew and loved the Lord. For a start I felt His Love for her – it would have been impossible otherwise even for me. Another clue is when Peter became bedridden, I would pass Joan's room on the left before I got to his further down on the right. So, if Joan was in her room I would pop in before going into Peter. The same **** language usually greeted my 'hello' and my reply that I loved her was followed usually by silence. On occasions, as I was going on down to Peter, Joan's town crier voice belted out enthusiastically a rendition of 'All things bright and beautiful....." or another of the well-known hymns, and she loved singing them. When I put two and two together, I knew that she had been a committed Christian and had loved the Lord. Also, that dementia had tried to destroy her and her faith. And I look back now and thank God for the privilege of knowing her and the way He used me regularly to confirm in her spirit that He loved her. Dementia may destroy the mind but cannot destroy the spirit of a person. When we give our lives to Jesus Christ we are born again of the Spirit of God; when our body dies and is buried, our spirit never dies but leaves the body and goes up to heaven.

CHAPTER 21

GO FOR IT PETE!

PETER ALWAYS LIKED to walk even well into dementia. He liked walking the dogs with me over Hothfield Common – a very large area of heathland outside Ashford… woods and open areas, streams and ponds. For years there has been some Highland cattle and a group of Konik ponies from Poland; the latter had hair growing thick and long in winter, even over their hooves because they came originally from a severe winter climate. When that was too much for Peter, Christine and I adapted the walks to places that were flat with gardens and small woods, and a café and a loo! This eventually was cut down to the occasional walk from the home down the road to a small wood below. Then we scaled down to a family cream tea at Dobbie's. Pete had always loved a cream tea. And a couple of years running we managed a few summer-time visits to our bungalow – he loved sitting in the summer house under the big cherry tree. But gradually by the end of the first few years at the home, all the visiting was the three of us visiting him. It was just a gradual limitation that is part and parcel of this long goodbye of dementia.

But at the home Peter was always walking around the building – mainly inside in winter, but a lot around the garden in the warmer months and sunny days. There were a lot of activities provided for the residents and some were where family members were invited.

The first INCIDENT they told us of was when Peter went missing; they searched high and low in the building and got very concerned. Then someone coming to work walked in with Peter. He was going for a walk out of the car park, probably down to the woods he had been taken on walks to previously. When they got him inside and checked him out, they asked him how he had got outside. Another member of staff standing beside him saw ink marks on one of his hands. He looked more closely and there was the four number code for using the lifts. Peter had watched someone put the code in, went for a biro and wrote the code on the palm of his hand, used it on the lift on the top floor, got himself down to the ground floor and walked out the front door! My thoughts went back to the cognitive test he had at the hospital and the banker in him excelled, remembering eighteen numbers spoken to him. When the manager rang to tell me (they always informed me of an incident), I sounded concerned, but to myself I was smiling and silently thought: 'Good on you, Pete! Go for it!' PS to that – they started changing the lift code number regularly!!

INCIDENT 2: Peter loved getting out in the garden at the home, so when the weather was warm enough for gardening activities Pete was out there raring to go. Even in the winter, Chris, Ian and I visiting together at weekends, would wrap him up warm and take him for a walk in the garden, sit on the garden seat round the back, and walk him back and in for a cuppa.

One day Pete was helping plant cuttings on the top of the front slope of the garden; he had helped the leader get the wheelbarrow with some cuttings and topsoil up to the top of the slope. The idea was to plant something there that would grow up and bush out a bit, to hide the view of vehicles passing when coming off the large roundabout next to the home, and give more privacy to the residents of the home.

Peter had observed more than they gave him credit for, for one late afternoon the manager had a frantic phone call from a friend of hers, who was waiting at the traffic lights nearest to the home; she happened to be a close friend of the manager and rang her personal phone number, shouting: "Get into your garden quick; there's an elderly gentleman astride the fence just feet away from the traffic lights. Any moment now he will be on the road and there could be a nasty accident..." Apparently Pete had used the wheelbarrow as a support to mount the fence!

The manager called the ground floor nurse on duty, and they flew through the activities room and out the door into the garden. And there was Pete, just as the phone caller had described; he was manoeuvring himself to drop down the other side. They shouted to him to be careful and said they would help him down safely. With a dementia brain I think he simply took it that they were helping down the way he was going. They managed to get him down and back inside without too much protest, and when he was out of sight another member of staff put the wheelbarrow safely away. It was never left out in the garden in the summer season after that!

INCIDENT 3: Early one morning about 6.30am there was the shrill sound of the fire alarm. It is normal practice I believe for the staff on duty to close the fire doors at night. If not, fire doors shut when the fire alarm went off, dividing the whole building on all floors into sections, designed to restrict a fire to just a small part of the building. There was only a skeleton staff on overnight, with a qualified nurse on duty on each floor. The fire alarms were at the same point on each floor, probably about eight to ten yards from the nurse's desks. All had been quiet, and most folk would be asleep. Well, almost – the nurse on the top floor jumped up and looked down both corridors. And there was one person up – Peter Ross. He wasn't touching the fire alarm, but he was standing near it. The security doors on his corridor were firmly closed, and the fire alarm near to him was deafening to him. They may have changed the alarms by now, but I remember the glass front on it with the words BREAK glass.

There was a hive of activity, but for the time being they were mystified because the glass on the alarm near where Peter was standing had not been broken. It was manic. Procedure was to get everyone into the carpark. The manager was rung – she was suffering from a hangover, wasn't due in until after lunch, and didn't want to take any chances being caught drunk and driving. The priority, and other staff were contacted and asked to come in and help, was getting everyone out and into the car park.

When a member of staff went to unlock the front door, there was a problem. It wouldn't unlock. It appeared that the fire alarm had affected this unwelcome bit of security. By the time they had got that sorted, they had also solved, in the top floor, the mystery of the fire alarm going off without the glass being broken. The nurse on duty knew Peter very well, approached him to check he was okay, chatted to him, and casually asked him if he knew how the fire alarm could be set off. He willingly showed her that all you had to do was put a finger under the lower edge of the glass and lift it up. The rest was obvious. Peter had done just this and simply pressed the button. Whether he, at his stage of dementia, was aware that he had set the alarm off over the whole building is doubtful. But it did expose the problem of the alarm setting the front door sort of doubly locked, stopping anyone going out or coming in! So, Peter did them a favour, though giving him credit for uncovering that fault would be stretching reality beyond belief!

The manager was rung and told there was no rush, all sorted and to come into the office when she was due, and the changeover staff would explain, and everything was also recorded in the incident book!

CHAPTER 22

THE MOBILE YEARS UP TO 2017

THE **MOBILE YEARS** had nothing to do with phones, but mobility – Peter's mobility! And he certainly put in some mileage in the dementia Lodge. Right from the start he would be walking around the corridors, having a good look in rooms where doors were open, and I was told on more than one occasion that he followed the duty doctor into another resident's room. When told not to come in by the Lodge nurse accompanying the doctor on his rounds, Peter insisted that it was his job to help the doctor. Once again, as I had seen and learned with other residents, the job or position they had in their working lives would draw them into situations where briefly they would be acting out their past work. After leaving the banking world Peter spent the last years of his working life thoroughly enjoying a late career in nursing.

But Peter became a bit of a faller too. In the years after he retired, well before the years the dementia was recognised, he had the occasional TIA, otherwise known as a mini stroke, that would usually recover quickly without any apparent after affects.

The first one we knew of was one Sunday after a church service. Someone came to get me to say that the chap on door duty had seen Peter stop in his tracks, his eyes went blank, and he dropped his hymn book without realising, and started to tip forward. The chap caught Pete and told someone nearby to tell me that he had taken Pete straight to the local hospital. I followed as soon as I heard; they had fast tracked him in to see a doctor, who immediately diagnosed a TIA, and Peter had completely recovered from all visible symptoms by the time he was in with the doctor.

The doctor asked me some leading questions and I offered him the information that Peter snored loudly when asleep and there would be gaps when he stopped breathing. As a result, an appointment would be sent in the post for Peter to visit the respiratory clinic; and as a result of that a follow-up appointment and more specific tests were called for. Peter was diagnosed with 'sleep apnoea'. He was sent home with a mask to wear at night that was meant to feed his lungs with oxygen and help him to breathe normally. The first night he put it on as instructed, but he hated wearing it, took it off and refused to use it ever again.

So, the condition remained untreated, and in retrospect now it possibly was a contributary factor in Peter developing dementia, which was Peter's final diagnosis and was the end game of the long goodbye. And linked to all of this was the fact that Peter was becoming a faller. I remember Ian saying to me one day, that often when he visited his dad in the dementia care lodge, and he would simply go walkabout with Dad, that Dad would stop in his tracks and start to tip forwards. Ian would grab hold of his dad and in a minute or even less his eyes were focussing normally, and they would carry on their stroll around the corridors

Of course, over the five plus years that Peter was in the Lodge, there were many falls. Peter became known as a faller so more attention was given, and he would be walked back to his room by a member of staff, rather than being left alone to his own devices.

But the falls continued, and as Peter wore spectacles, when his head hit the floor, there were often cuts above and below his eyes, on his cheeks, and on his nose. I was always informed and drove up to casualty in the car and after he was patched up, I drove him back to the home.

But it never was as simple as that sounds because of the lengthy wait in A&E for the obligatory tests for head injuries – blood tests, x-rays, and CT scans were the minimum, and proved very stressful for someone with advanced dementia. When he had a fall one afternoon when I was visiting him, and the injury was above his eye, I tried to persuade the Lodge nurse to do a 'butterfly stitch' on it using a plaster. My dad had shown me how to do it. He learnt in World War 2, on a civil defence course, for working in the night shelters in case of night bombing raids by Germany. But no, the home couldn't take chances. So, the ambulance was called yet again and I followed in the car. We got to A&E at 4pm, and it was so busy there were no cubicles free and Peter was

118

put in a spare room on the way in the corridor, that was filled with ambulance men and trolleys all the way back to the outside where the ambulances were parked with customers also waiting to come in.

Christine joined me after her supper, and during our wait we were supplied with tea and biscuits. The mandatory tests took ages and Peter was fidgeting and at times aggressive, and the ambulance men helped distract him whilst they were in the long queue. We got back to the dementia home at midnight, and I thought – 'never again, enough is enough.'

The last straw was when I got a call to say that Peter had been found standing outside his bedroom door with blood pouring from a wound in his head, and splashes of blood down the door frame and on the floor. They patched him up and called for the ambulance They then called me. I got into the car and went up to the hospital.

I was relieved to see Peter was in a bed in A&E, and his head was swathed in a bandage covering a dressing that the ambulance man had put on him before putting him in the ambulance at the nursing home. A nurse was sitting with Peter, obviously very necessary, as he was throwing his legs over the sides of the bed, although the metal safety sides had been pulled up to full height to keep him in! I told the nurse she could go back to her duties and thanked her for looking after him until I came. I added that I hoped the doctor wouldn't be too long in the circumstances, and I would like to have a word with him. Both Peter's legs were dangling over the side again by now!

Five minutes, and the doctor was at the bedside, introducing himself, shaking my hand, asking me what I would like to say. I confirmed I was both Peter's wife and his Power-of-Attorney. I explained the multiple falls and visits to A&E, and the long waits, the last one lasting eight hours. I re-affirmed what was obvious – that Peter had advanced dementia, that I would take full responsibility for him and said please no x-rays, no blood tests, and no CT scans. I knew this was the line of action and responsibility that he usually must take. "But look at him," I said.

He smiled and looked so relieved and said he would have a look at the wound, which he did. It was a sharp, clear cut on the side of Peter's head that had pretty well stopped bleeding. He said he would dress the wound and cover it. He said that yes, it is normal procedure to do all the tests that I named, and indeed the wait to get them all done can be lengthy. He thanked me for being so clear in my request and he would expedite my request. I agreed and thanked him.

Peter was back in the Lodge in less than two hours. I had also made another decision in my head but told no one and slept on it prayerfully. Next day when I visited the Lodge, the senior nurse was at her desk and was just the person I wanted to speak to, and so I went up to her. Firstly, I explained what I had said to the consultant the day before, and she was in absolute agreement and thanked me for my courage. So then, from that place I spoke specifically to her that I wanted a DNR notice on Peter's medical notes.

She was already nodding in agreement as I explained that after the many experiences in recent months, after falls, of being with Peter in A&E, and the decision I made with the doctor the day before. I knew that his dementia was advancing at such a rate, and it was time, as both his wife and POA, to protect him from any unnecessary suffering. The resuscitation process that is performed on someone whose heart has stopped, often results in broken ribs and more suffering. When it is Peter's time to go, I want him to go, in his own bed, gently and quietly, and hopefully I will be there with him, though I have come to realise over the last few years that many folk breathe their last when the person sitting with them leaves the room!

She agreed totally and this subject relating to Peter had been discussed with senior staff, including the manager, only a couple of days before. We were by now well into 2017, and Peter was now spending each day partly in the lounge and dining room dozing or having his meals with a little more help eating; or on his bed if he wanted to. An additional piece of equipment was added – a sensor mat beside his bed, because he was found fallen out of bed and not able to get up, and now if he fell out of bed or even got out onto the sensor mat a warning sound would alert someone on duty and his room number would flash up. From this time onwards someone would

121

always now be walking him to the dining room and back.

The writing of this is vividly reminding me of the downward slope to eventual death that is every dementia sufferer's future; even today, four years later, there is still no known cure for this disease. And I do emphasise 'DISEASE' again. Continuing Care Assessment was still assessing Peter NOT having a disease at this stage but a social condition.

Up until now, Peter, like most of us, was under NHS care whenever needed. But the moment he got so advanced and ill with dementia, he could no longer be safely looked after at home and had to go into a nursing home for dementia sufferers, paying £5,000 fees per month at the age of 82 years! That's no criticism of the home, just of the broken system of our health service that was in earlier years admired all over the world.

Mid-July 2017, Peter had quickly become bedridden and was now spending £5,700 monthly for his care. He would be 86 years old next birthday. The doctor was called and happened to arrive when I was visiting Peter. Whilst the nurse tidied his bed the doctor drew me aside and said there was nothing further she could do for him, and had authorized the three medicines needed for end-of-life patients. She squeezed my arm and left.

Next day Chris and I went in to see Peter and the nurse in charge, to discuss things that were very much on our mind.

Peter was dozing, so the nurse beckoned us outside. We sat in the sheltered, glassed outdoor area two doors from his room. She told us that the Royal College of Nursing end-of-life protocol for residents was to treat that patient as having three days to live.

The manager also contacted Continuing Care and they would ring back and make an appointment.

CHAPTER 23

THE BEGINNING OF THE END

S O, THE END-OF-LIFE protocol included three medicines in place, authorized by the doctor to be given to Peter for pain, agitation, and to reduce fluid increase in the lungs if and when needed.

Next day, as mentioned earlier, a very pleasant lady from Continuing Care arrived and I was invited to attend. She had been down to see Peter before I arrived. One of the nurses joined us at her request and we started an assessment. About five minutes into it, she called a halt to the assessment, saying she had visited Peter before the assessment, and now she asked the nurse if she agreed with her, that Peter was so advanced that it was a waste of time to continue, and Peter should be awarded Continuing Care immediately. Without hesitation the nurse agreed. Using her laptop this lovely lady set up the whole decision online and all three of us were able to sign. I was amazed – I didn't realise computers were so clever! She confirmed that from this day Peter was no longer paying for his care. Wow, just like that! A weight fell off my shoulders. And the next morning at 8.30am I was rung by a charming man from senior management of

Continuing Care to confirm that Peter would no longer be paying for his care.

Things were moving quickly; the logjam was gone!

Next an 'end-of-life' bed was ordered and was quickly in place. What a mechanical whizz of a machine that was – both sides could be put up or down, for staff to turn him regularly, wash him all over and clean him and change nappies. Switched on all the time in inflating and deflating mode so that one part of his body after another was on a gentle wave, giving relief to all weight-bearing parts of his body in turn.

And I must say that this piece of equipment together with the wonderful work of the carers had great results. The end-of-lifetime of three days in July 2017 went on for over another seven months until Peter died in March 2018, and he never had any sort of bedsores ever. Amazing and thanks and congratulations to the staff who regularly repeated this standard of body care for all those long months.

He ate and drank less and less and as his swallowing mechanism began to fail, they took great care in feeding him, liquidizing his food first and later resorting to a variety of plain yoghurts. Everything was recorded on a food and fluid chart, and occasionally some days had 'nil' written on it. One afternoon I came in and went down to his room. I heard a quiet woman's voice, so I just peeped around the edge of the door frame and saw one of the young Thai girls feeding Peter. He looked very relaxed and so did she, holding a teaspoon of yoghurt, waiting for him to be ready. Sometimes he swallowed, other times he didn't. And she wiped his chin gently when there was a bit of a dribble. As I watched the sense of peace grew between them and touched me deeply too. Then as she smiled at him, I heard her quietly say: "I love you Peter Ross." Totally taken by surprise, my tears welled up. What a 'Carer' with a capital C! And I quietly turned and went back down the corridor to the dining room, and enjoyed a cup of tea, with the peace lingering.

I was now in the habit of coming to visit Pete most days, sometimes twice, again in the evening after supper, a lovely peaceful time. I was grateful for friends who visited too, but a special mention of Sylvia and Derek who for a long time had been visiting Peter regularly every week and more often when Pete was put in 'end-of-life', and when 'the beast from the east' February 2018 weather began to thaw, these two friends were able to come in every day the last few days.

CHAPTER 24

THE HULLO AND GOODBYE BLESSINGS

THERE WERE TWO THINGS I started to do every time I visited Peter in those last few months. The first was to stop saying goodbye to him when I left. In the earlier years there he would struggle with carers when I got into the lift. Then when I lingered and sat quietly talking and we both were very relaxed, and I rested my hand gently on his, he would close his eyes and nod off, and I quietly left.

Fast forward to Peter in the end-of-life bed; he was often vague when I went into his room, looking blankly at me, and anxious when I got up to say goodbye. I had heard folk say about their spouse or parent that he or she wasn't their mum or dad or wife or husband anymore. I of course understood exactly what they meant; many were so broken by this that they just couldn't visit anymore.

I thought deeply about these things but came to a convinced and rooted-in conclusion that Peter would always be my husband until he breathed his last breath and God took him home. This conviction set me off on two practical exercises that were the fruit of this solid conviction. The first was when I visited and entered his room. I would go to the foot of his bed and if he was awake, he would look blankly at me, which was more frequent as the days came and went. And not only that, his mouth was by now never closed, but wide open. I would speak to him clearly and slowly: "Peter Ross, this is Sue your wife come to see you. You've only got one wife Peter Ross, and that's me, and I am coming to give you a big kiss."

My strategy would only work if I could get his mouth to close, because it was now permanently open, and open very wide with gunge in it, that the carers did clear several times a day. So, as I moved closer repeating who I was and that I was coming to give him a big kiss, I would say: "Here I am, this is Sue!"

I gently placed my index finger just under his ear, and repeated: "I'm coming!" And slowly drew my finger from his ear across his cheek towards his mouth. He got it first time, and rapidly pouted his lips in anticipation! He got it first time… no practice needed! All I had to do was follow the same ritual with him whenever I visited him, and he always pouted his lips at the same rate right up to the day he died.

What major lesson did I take from that? Well, I have heard so many folks struggling with the decline in their nearest and dearest not knowing who they were when they visited, that they couldn't cope with visiting anymore, being too upset, and how often I heard the broken cry that the dementia sufferer didn't know who their, mother, father, husband, wife, were.

I cracked that with one simple ritual, after a lot of prayer, and I offer that to folk reading this, to take hold of it and use it when visiting close relatives dying with dementia. Take the initiative and you and your sick relative will both be blessed.

The second strategy was saying goodbye to Peter after visiting him through those last final months, in a way that didn't distress him. Back to prayer again seeking God's wisdom. Yes! So simple... why didn't I think of that before? Well, although He is profound in all His ways, He often has a simple answer to our problems. We often struggle away with a problem, chew over the ifs and buts and end up with a complicated solution that rarely works.

But taking God's lead, I did this when it was time to leave Peter. My way had been to stand up and say that I must go because the dogs need a walk, or I must go to Sainsbury's on my way home. Result – an anxious husband who of course didn't want me to go.

God's leading once I asked Him – I stayed sitting close to Peter, holding his hand: "Peter, before I leave, I want to pray with you; is that okay with you?" I hadn't moved and was still holding his hand. He nodded. I lifted my other hand and laid it on his forehead and closed my eyes. I immediately spoke over him two Scriptures that came to mind – one from the New Testament of the Bible, then one from the Old Testament. "Peter, may the Peace of God which surpasses all understanding keep your heart and mind in the knowledge of God and His

Son, Jesus Christ. And may God bless you and keep you and make His face to shine upon you and give you His Peace. Amen."

All quiet; I opened my eyes and looking into his face, my dear husband's eyes were closed, and his steady gentle breathing told me he was fast asleep. I lifted my hand off his head and quietly left the room with a mixture of joy and peace in my own heart, causing tears to fall in gratitude to our God.

CHAPTER 25

THE PEACE BEYOND ALL UNDERSTANDING

I **CONTINUED** to use the hello and goodbye blessings on what had become daily visits right up to his last day. They never failed and more so that lovely Peace started to grow and was touching others in the team.

Christine and I had some months before I booked a holiday end January into February 2018. About a month before the senior nurse assured us that Peter, though so advanced, was quite stable, and encouraged us to take the break. About ten days before she suggested that we postpone our break. So, I rang Saga and as usual they were very helpful, cancelled the holiday at no extra charge and passed on the team's condolences, and said to feel free to book another break when we were ready.

As is usual I always make lists for packing suitcase and hand luggage, at least two weeks before, and so ten days before I was well ahead with my packing.

Then came the weather forecast – what was being called 'the beast from the east' was moving under strong winds down from the Arctic. As the anticyclone came south the winds heading in our direction in Kent turned to us from the east, so the Russian winter was rapidly moving toward us.

I knew I would not be able to get up my one hundred metre driveway and onto the road in my car once it snowed. And our road is narrow and doesn't get salted in winter. So snap decision: I got holiday clothes out of my hand luggage and put warmer clothes in with my already full washbag! The dogs had already gone on their Barking Mad holidays. So, I was free to go down to the Lodge with my holdall: "Could I have a room please?" Of course, no hesitation from the manager, who showed me to a spare room just a few yards from Peter's. What a relief; I was in the right place and peace settled in my heart. And I rang Chris and told her where I was.

The next day Chris arrived with the necessary luggage, and they found a room for her too. Brilliant! We were fed and watered gratis, and the chef was good, very good!

In the days before when visiting Peter more and more staff would come in and comment on the peace they saw in Peter, and asked what it was. I simply said that Peter loved Jesus, and it was His Presence in the room; and that in the Bible it says Jesus is the Prince of Peace. And so, it continued with Chris and I living in this dementia care home for the last week of Peter's life. That Peace grew – certainly even as I sat and watched Peter's body shrinking to nothing but skin and bone, lying in a foetal position, eyes usually closed and not speaking or moving – THAT PEACE GREW.

The second morning there the doctor from the surgery came to visit. She stood at the bottom of the bed and pointed at Peter and said: "That is a miracle!" I nodded as she looked at me.

She continued very quietly: "Yes, a miracle; you see, as with all end-of-life residents, the senior nurse legally needs permission from a doctor to have ready to use three drugs to ease pain, agitation, and to control the increase of fluid in the lungs." She pointed again at Peter and said: "He now has no need for any of those drugs. He is so far advanced now that he will simply and quietly stop breathing." I couldn't have wished for any more; thank you Jesus.

Sometimes Chris and I were both in the room with Peter; on other occasions it was just one of us. Chris would, as the weather eased up, go to Sainsbury's for a few items either of us needed, or meet with a friend for coffee and a natter. I would go out for walks or check on my bungalow and touch base with my lovely neighbours when the snow melt had started.

I had never met the night duty staff, so it was a lovely surprise to have the senior night shift nurse to come into Peter's room, on my first night there, when I was sitting in the armchair by his bed. With a bit of an accent, she enquired: "Are you Sue?" I nodded.

She continued, pointing at Peter: "I want to say something about that."

"What?" I enquired expectantly.

"That peace on him… it's lovely!"

"Well, he's a Christian who loves Jesus; it's the Peace of God."

She looked at me. "It's wonderful…" And then pointing at me, she said: "And it's on you too!"

My heart leapt with Joy, and she turned and left in response to someone in the corridor calling her. Later when I left Peter to go to my room, I saw her down the corridor, all quiet, having finished the evening drugs round. So, I walked up to her. "Hi again; that accent of yours – where is it from?"

"Romania," she smiled.

I looked her in the eye and said, "And you are a born-again Christian as well, aren't you?"

"Oh yes," she said. And we said goodnight and parted with a big hug.

That's family, a stranger in one moment and then a sister that will endure way beyond this life. And in this last week in the Lodge, God was showering me with gifts of love, peace, joy and grace.

One evening I checked with Chris if it was okay for me to have an evening at the bungalow. I picked up a ready meal with pudding at Sainsbury's on the way. I put the central heating on and sat watching the telly and enjoying my meal. I didn't intend falling asleep and the phone ringing made me jump.

It was Christine, and I can still hear her quiet voice saying simply: "He's gone."

I immediately replied: "I'm coming."

One moment asleep, the next I jumped to my feet, and it hit me. For possibly five minutes, I don't know, time seemed to stand still, the shock hit me first... and yet it wasn't a shock. It was the long goodbye finished... full stop. And I started to howl – to me I sounded like a wild animal; and I was walking round and round in small circles in my living room just howling like a wild animal in acute pain.

It subsided and a quiet gentle peace returned.

My head got into gear and I put warm clothes on and walked up the drive to the road where I had left my car. It took me about three minutes to get to the Lodge as there was no traffic on the road, because of the snow still on the ground. But as I drove a weight lifted off me and I had a gentle mix of peace and joy. I kept repeating, 'Thank you God, thank you God, thank you God. Dementia couldn't hold onto him; it had to let him go, and you have taken him home, thank you, thank you.'

By this time, I was driving into the Lodge. I parked, got in using the code, and went up in the lift. All quiet – well past everyone's bedtime. Outside Peter's room I was met by the senior nurse on duty, a teddy bear of a man whom I had known for a long time. He wrapped his arms around me and held me tight. He said, "Are you alright?

"Yes," I said quietly, and he pointed to Peter's room and said: "Chris is in there."

I opened the door and went in. Chris was standing back a bit beside the bed, so without saying anything I went straight to the bed and looked on my husband's face. He was at peace. I leaned forward, put my hand on the side of his head and kissed him on his forehead, and said my final goodbye. I felt relieved that he was still warm, and turned to Chris to say so. She put her hands out and we held each other tight, allowing the tears to flow freely.

We went out to the nurse. He said he had called the funeral parlour. Where possible it was best to get the deceased taken away at night so that people weren't around to be upset. So, we arranged to come back the next morning to clear Peter's room, which we did.

Jesus said: "I am the Resurrection and the life. He who believes in Me will live, even though he dies; and whoever lives and believes in me will never die. Do you believe this?"

John 11:25-26

Printed in Great Britain
by Amazon

76566750R10088